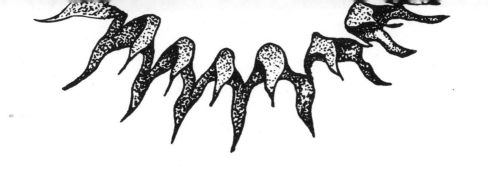

Ann Wigmore's

Recipes for Longer Life

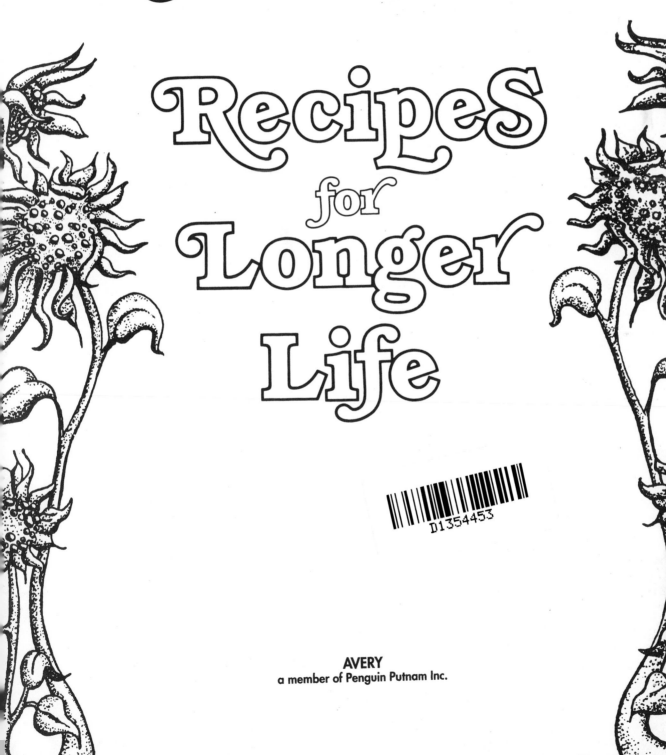

AVERY
a member of Penguin Putnam Inc.

The medical and health procedures in this book
are based on the training, personal experiences, and
research of the author. Because each person and
situation is unique, the author and publisher urge
the reader to check with a qualified health professional
before using any procedure where there is any question
as to its appropriateness.

The publisher does not advocate the use of any
particular diet and exercise program, but believes the
information presented in this book should be available
to the public.

Because there is always some risk involved, the
author and publisher are not responsible for any adverse
effects or consequences resulting from the use of any
of the suggestions, preparations, or procedures in this
book. Please do not use the book if you are unwilling to
assume the risk. Feel free to consult a physician or
other qualified health professional. It is a sign of
wisdom, not cowardice, to seek a second or third
opinion.

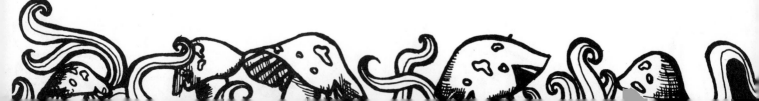

Contents

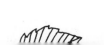
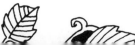

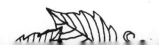

A DIFFERENT APPROACH TO THE VITAMIN QUESTION

There has been more research work done on vitamins than any other component of food, and yet the basic facts of vitamins are almost lost upon both researchers and laymen.

It is necessary to recognize "living forces" as separate and apart from materialistic concepts. It is impossible to analyze or separate out vitamins. The vitamins are something immaterial -- a "living force." Foods rich in vitamins, such as wheat grass or carrots, take on the "living forces" so that the "living forces" are integral with the wheat grass and carrots but cannot be separated from them. The "living forces" may be lost but cannot be separated out.

What is the main source of this "living force"? The main source is the sun. We think of the sun's rays as light rays, but in reality many different types of rays come into the world from the sun, and these are not all visible to us. The infrared rays and ultraviolet rays are examples.

Foods rich in vitamin A, such as oils and seeds, are those which are rich in "warmth." Warmth derives from the sun -- mostly from the infrared rays of the sun.

Foods rich in vitamin B are those rich in "order" such as the husks of wheat berries or rice and the peels of fruit. Order derives from the ultraviolet rays of the sun.

Foods rich in vitamin C are those rich in "light" such as green leaves (wheat grass). Light derives from the visible rays of the sun.

Vitamin D is in another category. The best way to describe vitamin D is to relate an experiment with pigeons which had the oil glands under their tails removed. They developed rickets, the prime vitamin D deficiency disease. When preening their feathers, the pigeons could no longer oil their feathers to allow the sun to irradiate the oil into vitamin D, with resultant absorption of the irradiated oil into the birds' skins. Undoubtedly our best vitamin D is the vitamin D we ourselves can properly absorb through our skin from the rays of the sun. My personal belief and practice is to expose a reasonable amount of my skin to the sun whenever conveniently possible.

Paradoxically, the warmth, light, and air which impart the "living forces" to growing foods will destroy them after they have been harvested. Take hay, for example, which is livestock's chief sources of complete vitamins. A farmer will store his hay, protecting it as much as possible from light, heat, and moving air current. Years ago there were dairies which bottled milk in amber-colored bottles to protect the milk from light. The milk was to be kept refrigerated and sealed except when poured for use. The same principles apply to all "living food," once harvested. The food should be protected as much as possible from warmth, light, and air.

Harvey C. Lisle

A WORD FROM HARVEY G. LISLE
TECHNICAL ADVISOR TO ANN WIGMORE

I graduated in 1937 from Ohio State University, where I had majored in chemistry. After getting out of the U.S. Air Force, I worked as a chemist for an agricultural laboratory (the Brookside Laboratory) where I tested soils and animal fodder, and subsequently I worked as a food technologist. At the same time, I took up my avocation of testing food for human consumption.

My chief diagnostic tool for testing foodstuffs is "paper chromotography." Paper chromatograms are mediums for telling whether or not a food has been raised organically/naturally; whether it is full of life forces or devoid of such forces. While this testing method gives only basic answers, these are basic answers essential to a "grass roots movement" of people interested in a more natural lifestyle.

Ann Wigmore, with her lay organization, the Hippocrates Health Institute, is a prime example of a person needing help ordinarily unavailable from any professional source. I agreed to help her in those areas where I felt qualified. Such help has always been rendered out of love for humanity and not out of love for remuneration.

One of the keys to Ann Wigmore's program is the raising of wheatgrass and the consumption of wheatgrass chlorophyll. The growing of wheatgrass is relatively simple and can be carried out by anyone who desires to do so, regardless of whether at Ann Wigmore's Mansion, at home, in a desert region, or even on travels. Although raising wheatgrass is simple, there are a few fundamental rules which must be followed if the grass is to be of value. With the help of my experience and testing methods, we were able to devise with Dr. Ann what we think is the optimum method for raising the kind of wheatgrass which incorporates the highest grade of chlorophyll, vitamins, minerals, and enzymes.

The next step was to determine whether the fresh wheatgrass juice should be drunk immediately or whether it could be made in advance and then stored in the refrigerator for a few hours or any other length of time. Although we had a good idea of what the answer would be, it took a little research to arrive at a fairly definite time span. The answer was as follows: for the maximum benefit, the freshly-extracted juice must be consumed within fifteen minutes of its preparation. Research done by other scientists on a variety of juices (including wheatgrass juice) shows that a median time lapse of only seven minutes is recommended for full benefits. We are all, therefore, in full agreement that a freshly-extracted juice of fresh living produce must be drunk almost immediately.

Ann Wigmore asked me to formulate a salad that would be complete in food values, including proteins. This research involved not laboratory facilities, but books and tables which gave such diverse information as amino acid values, calories, percentage of fat or carbohydrates, life energy (resistance), etc. Such a salad was formulated with the provision that if a person was still hungry or had a craving after eating, that person was allowed to satisfy his/her appetite by supplementation with other vegetarian food.

There were a number of what I would call minor problems which Dr. Ann asked me to address. For example, almost everyone likes watermelons, but almost no one eats the white meat of the inner rind which borders the red fruit. Analysis proved the white portion to be very rich in nutrients. Tests on family and friends confirmed that the white meat is very easily digestible -- so the conclusion is obvious. The taste of the white meat is not ojbectionable; the only consideration is that this portion is harder to chew than the inner red fruit. Therefore, for the sake of health and the strengthening of much-needed will power, go ahead and eat it for all-around benefit. As is widely known today, the minerals and vitamins, as well as the enzymes, of all fruits and vegetables are located predominantly in rinds and skins and immediately underneath them.

Another major key to Dr. Ann Wigmore's Health Program is enzyme-rich fermented foods: seed sauces and cheeses and a drink called Rejuvelac. She never told me how she came to develop this most beneficial beverage, but she told me how it is made and asked me to find out all I could about it. I found that Rejuvelac shows immediate good results. It is simply a drink of fermented cereal grains. Fermentation of grains creates a high enzymatic activity, which is the basic essential of Rejuvelac. Human digestion is dependent upon enzymatic activity, so those people in ill health or with poor digestion benefit especially from drinking this very slightly sour liquid.

While Dr. Ann Wigmore's main thrust is restoration of good health for those who lack it (especially those afflicted with grave and painful malfunctions like cancer), she has other allied interests. One of these is the health of our pets. Another is the improvement of school lunches.

This pretty much concludes the majority of projects we have carried out for Dr. Ann Wigmore. It is my conviction that healing is still more of an art than a science. Ann Wigmore has the background, conviction, and talents to carry out her healing program successfully. I am pleased that I could add my small talents to help her along her chosen path.

Harvey Lisle
Norwalk, Ohio - September, 1980

PROFILE OF DR. ANN WIGMORE

Dr. Ann founded the Hippocrates Health Institute in Boston to share her Living Food Program with the world. It is the home base of the Hippocrates World Health Organization, founded by Dr. Ann in 1970 and which is now growing rapidly with centers in Michigan and Bombay, India. The HWHO is an educational, humanitarian, non-profit organization devoted to the physical, mental, and spiritual development of mankind through a living, uncooked, diet. Students come from all over the world to learn the Living Food Program, and return home equipped to teach to others the techniques they have learned. With its emphasis on sprouting, fermenting, composting, and living food, there is no other program like it in the world.

Ann has repeatedly shown that the body will heal itself of any illness when it is given Living Food Nourishment. Sprouts, wheatgrass, seeds, grains, indoor greens, fermented sauces and uncooked fruits and vegetables -- that is, all living foods which are easily digestible and wonderfully nutritious -- form the staple of her Living Food Program. These living foods have been shown by Dr. Ann to provide the body with everything it needs for optimum health, harmony, and vitality.

During her long and loving service to humanity (twenty-seven years), she has received numerous honors and awards for her outstanding work in the field of health and human nutrition. In 1971, The Nobel Prize Foundation (Royal Laplander Academy of Science) in Europe presented her with a Recognition Award for work in the Field of Youthfulness and for Efforts in Regeneration of Human Cells and Tissues; in 1978, Dr. Ann was made Lady Ann Wigmore by the Kingdom of the Netherlands which presented her with its highest award, the Order of Chivalry, for "distinguished achievement and noble deeds" in recognition of her outstanding work in the field of health and human ecology. In 1979, she was presented with a Cancer Victory Award by the Arlin J. Brown Information Center "in appreciation for saving numerous lives... ."

As far back as 1975, the House of Representatives of the Commonwealth of Massachusetts had awarded her with a citation for "exemplary development of food self-sufficiency through the wise use of natural resources." Dr. Ann had donated five years of teaching workshops in the Boston area to high schools and colleges. These workshops on sprouting, healing, and soil composting are very popular. She co-lectured for many years with her friend and colleage, Dr. Paul Dudley White, the famous heart specialist.

Ann has traveled extensively around the world promoting her Living Food Program. Between 1977 and 1979, she traveled to India three times. There she opened seven health restoration camps, lectured at the Medical Research Hospital, and opened a HWHO center in Bombay. There, as in America, thousands of ailing people were helped to health by her program of living food, sprouting, and colon cleansing. While in India, Dr. Ann also published four books, among them You Are Your Own Healer.

During August of 1980, Dr. Ann spent ten days in Finland where she was warmly received. While there, she generated considerable excitement because of her program; as a result, a number of significant events are now happening. Her books are going to be translated into Finnish, among many other languages.

As more and more people become educated about living foods and made aware of Nature's laws, they will begin to experience the power and grade behind Hippocrates' words, "Let food by thy medicine."

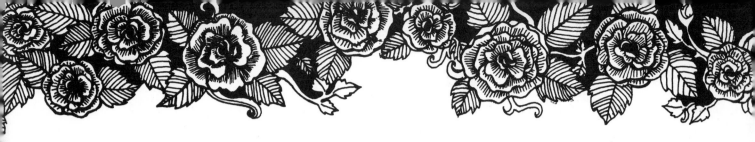

DEDICATION

To human angels everywhere who have become aware that living food
is the key not only to health and reduction of living costs in these
times of inflation, but also helpful in reducing the consumption of
energy and, more important, reducing the time needed to prepare meals.
Instead of spending three hours over the stove cooking and destroying
the life force in foods, one need spend a maximum of only one hour to
prepare the nourishment that God created. This living food cookbook
is also a means of survival and will provide guidelines for the pre-
vention and overcoming of sickness and old age.

These souls that have become human angels have taken it upon themselves to be examples. I would like to comment on their courage --
their courage to move into the change despite resistance encountered
from their family and friends -- and perhaps from society. I dedicate
this book to them because of their fortitude and faith in Nature
and God; their awakening desire to help themselves and their families
and friends (when they become ready to be helped); their interest in
helping humanity as a whole.

It has been a great privilege for me to work with these human angels
and to watch them grow and improve, not only physically and mentally,
but also spiritually, as they move into this New Age, through Nature's
and God's way -- by living food. So I want to say that these people
deserve my dedication as an encouragement to them to continue to join
my long-standing efforts to make a better world, the results of which
I begin to see manifested everywhere.

Again, let me say -- with my heart full of gratitude and love, and my
dedication -- that we will proceed until we have changed the whole
of humanity and its attitude toward caring, especially caring for
Nature, for one's body, for one's pets, for all of creation which
humankind has so unknowingly neglected. For your love through service,
I say, thank you, thank you.

Ann Wigmore, D.D., N.D.

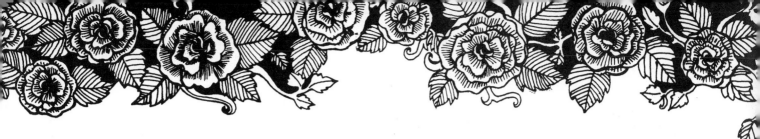

FOREWORD

The idea for the Recipe Book grew from a desire to share with others the knowledge of how easily raw food meals are prepared, how delicious they are, and how readily they can fit into any diet -- no matter what else that diet may include. This new edition appears at a time when there is great general interest in health. Those of you who share this interest will realize that by preparing these meals, you are promoting your health and that of your families -- for all the ingredients proposed are those belonging to Mother Nature herself.

Dr. Ann Wigmore's program of living foods has brought me great benefits and I'd like to help bring those benefits to you. The work accomplished at the Hippocrates Institute would not be possible without the hard work and vision of Dr. Ann. Her presence -- seen or unseen -- is felt throughout the Mansion as a beautiful example to us all. This book is also an expression of the loving hands, hearts, and spirits of all who have put their energy into the Hippocrates kitchen and who have provided in so many ways for the physical and spiritual welfare of those who come to the Mansion. What each Hippocrates' staff member gives is unique.

This book is the expression of their spirit and of the loving dedication and energy of Dr. Ann.

Ruth Rogers, M.D.

INTRODUCTION

Hippocrates, the Father of Medicine, taught that live food could restore and maintain vibrant health. Some four hundred years before the birth of Christ, he affirmed that "your food shall be your medicine, and your medicine shall be your food." Today, more than ever before, we should heed his words: modern living, with its cooked food, overstimulation, and destructive living habits, has made of our bodies clogged sewage systems (literally!).

I have stated continuously that only one sickness exists: malnutrition. Malnutrition manifests itself in various forms. It strikes the weakest part of the body, so that some persons may have cancer, heart trouble, or diabetes, while others are addicted to drugs or alcohol or become overweight. Still others are plagued by the mental disturbances which are so common in our country today.

We can allow our bodies to heal themselves, however, with a return to a more wholistic way of living, and particularly if we eat living foods. I have proved consistently that when deficiencies in the body are taken care of through organically-grown living food, we have the basis for a peaceful world. In this world there will no longer be the need to take alcohol or drugs or other harmful substances in an effort to escape from depression and anxieties.

We at the Hippocrates Health Institute in Boston are dedicated to making available to everyone the basic principles underlying easy, inexpensive ways to maintain health, vitality, and mental alertness. Visitors are offered practical, supervised experiences in sprouting, organic growing of greens, and food preparation and a simple diet of living food, plus instruction in the use of wheatgrass (chlorophyll) - and these form the basis of the art of self-healing.

The delicious and easily prepared meals suggested on the following pages have evolved from this program. RECIPES FOR LIFE are exactly that: recipes which consist of exclusively uncooked, living foods that contain life and truly impart life to the eaters thereof. Although the recipes are deceptively simple to prepare, inexpensive to purchase, incredibly delicious to the palate and beautiful to the eye -- do not be fooled: you are working with the most scientifically superior nutritional materials possible, those grown by Nature (God).

The cumulative effect of such menus will enable the lucky ones who enjoy "the complete meal salad," the miracle drink called "rejuvelac," the non-fattening, wholly natural cookies and candies, and many other wonderful dishes; to make great jumps in their energy levels and thus accomplish what they could not accomplish before. And -- who knows? -- they may be brought a little bit closer to becoming truly healthy, happy, and holy humans.

You might say, "You want me to believe that these recipes can perform such a miracle?" Our reply to you is, "Yes!" But you don't have to believe us! Ask the twenty-nine year old man who ran more than a hundred miles a day for weeks on end, until he crossed the continent of Australia in world-record time. He was a total raw-fooder. Ask members of the Pittsburgh Pirates baseball team, which won the World Series in 1979, what they think about the uncooked foods and fruit and vegetable juices added to their diets. These were added by a nutrition consultant who himself ran across America, doing fifty miles a day on less than 500 calories a day!

Even if you don't plan to run or bike across continents, you may well find that this book is for you. The delicious and easily prepared meals suggested on its pages have evolved from our self-healing program.

RECIPES FOR LIFE are for:

- Any mother who loves her husband and children and wants the very best for them including freedom from illness. Digestive problems and their resultant toxicity have soured many a marriage and have also been proven to contribute to problem behavior in children.

- Any nutritionally-oriented physicians or healers who would like to guide their patients to good health by way of "kitchen therapy" (a living foods program). They will find that each recipe is a true prescription for health.

- And for Everyman and Everywoman and Everychild who feels that there can be more to life and love in his or her life than presently experienced. The RECIPES FOR LIFE people say, "Eat as if your life depended on it -- it does!" Eat "God's greatest hits" -- whole foods, live foods, healthy foods, life-giving foods -- and then witness the incredible health benefits that these foods bestow upon us all!

Our experience at Hippocrates has shown that when our bodies are provided with the necessary nutritional elements, we need no longer fear degeneration, disease, or mental disorders. When we understand the basic care of the body and nourish it with living food, according to the principles of Nature's laws, we have taken the first step toward eliminating illness, mental and physical, and toward self-healing.

With the right combination of living foods, we can achieve and maintain the balance needed for us to overcome adverse conditions; we can achieve energy and youth and freedom from stress. We can, in short, achieve perfect health - mental, physical, and spiritual. It is to this aim, and with the vision of a peaceful, healthy world. that these recipes have been compiled.

Ann Wigmore, N.D., D.D.

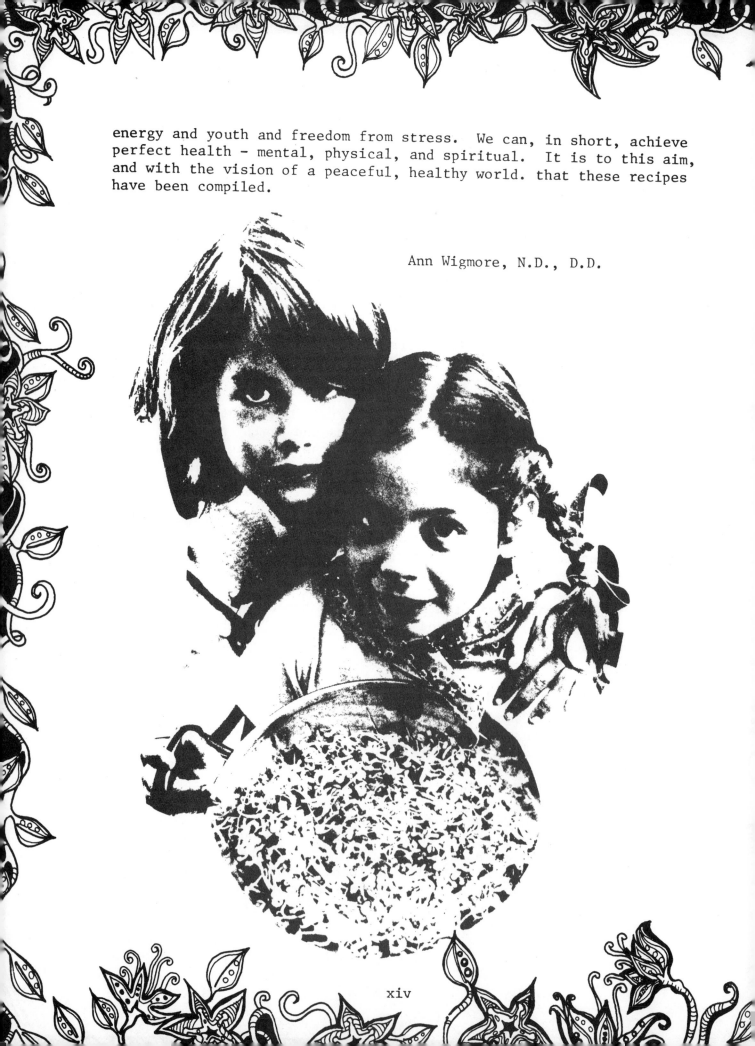

LIVING FOODS DEFINED
(An Excerpt from a letter to Ann Wigmore from Chemist Harvey Lisle)

To understand what organic food is, one must first understand the definition of organic soil, since food is the product of soil. I have read many definitions of organic soil and found that they tend to miss the main point. Organic soil has been defined as one in which no chemicals or poisons have been used and in which there is an adequate supply of humus or organic matter. This is correct, yet an important factor is missing: the key point in organic soil is balance.

To understand what is meant by balance, one must realize that all nature, all of life, is polarity. Polarities appear to be in opposition, but in reality control each other. Some easily-perceived polarities are: hot and cold, wet and dry, ... day and night, male and female ... If any one member of a polarity becomes too great at the expense of its opposite, then an unstable, unhealthy condition will persist until the two members of the polarities come back into balance ...

In grasping the concept of balance and its importance, we shall now consider what happens when a typical chemical fertilizer such as 6-24-12 is added to the soil (6% nitrogen - 24% phosphorous oxide - 12% potassium oxide). These ingredients are water soluble and absorbed much too rapidly by the soil. The soluble phosphorous and potassium tip the balance in their favor, and a true balance has been lost. Any food raised in that soil will not be in balance. Such unbalanced food will fill empty stomachs and sustain life but will not promote health.

To consider the attainment of a truly organic soil, the following points must be considered: the soil should be tested and brought into balance by earthworms and compost. .. Such a soil will then attract and be a home for many living organisms ... and will be a truly living soil.

Now, with a better understanding of what truly organic soil is, it will be a simpler matter to understand what an organic living food is. An organic living food is food which has been raised on an organic, balanced soil. Hopefully, it would be a well-balanced food with minerals, vitamins, and enzymes, all in balance. From a practical standpoint, sunshine, rain, and weather cannot be ignored in considering a balance ... However, knowing what it takes to develop an organic soil and what is required to raise organic food, we can strive for the best. ..[1]

---

1.   Your indoor garden can be a great help in this respect, as indoor gardeners can control the balance of nutrients in their soil. A.W.

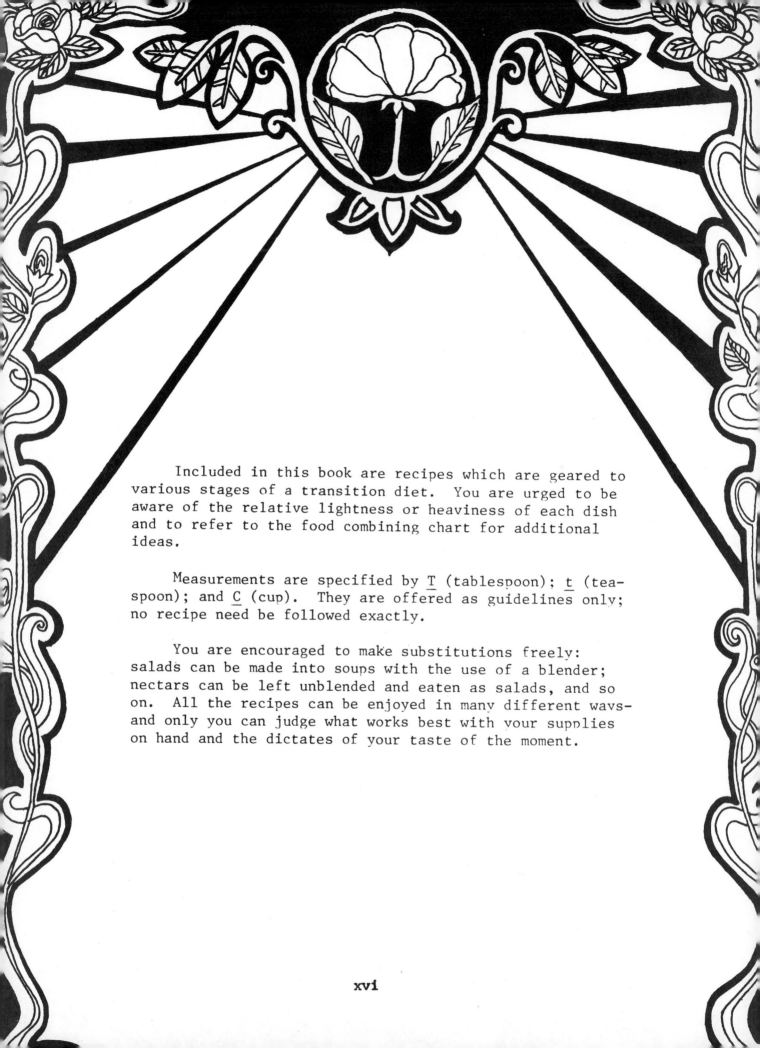

Included in this book are recipes which are geared to various stages of a transition diet. You are urged to be aware of the relative lightness or heaviness of each dish and to refer to the food combining chart for additional ideas.

Measurements are specified by $\underline{T}$ (tablespoon); $\underline{t}$ (teaspoon); and $\underline{C}$ (cup). They are offered as guidelines only; no recipe need be followed exactly.

You are encouraged to make substitutions freely: salads can be made into soups with the use of a blender; nectars can be left unblended and eaten as salads, and so on. All the recipes can be enjoyed in many different ways—and only you can judge what works best with your supplies on hand and the dictates of your taste of the moment.

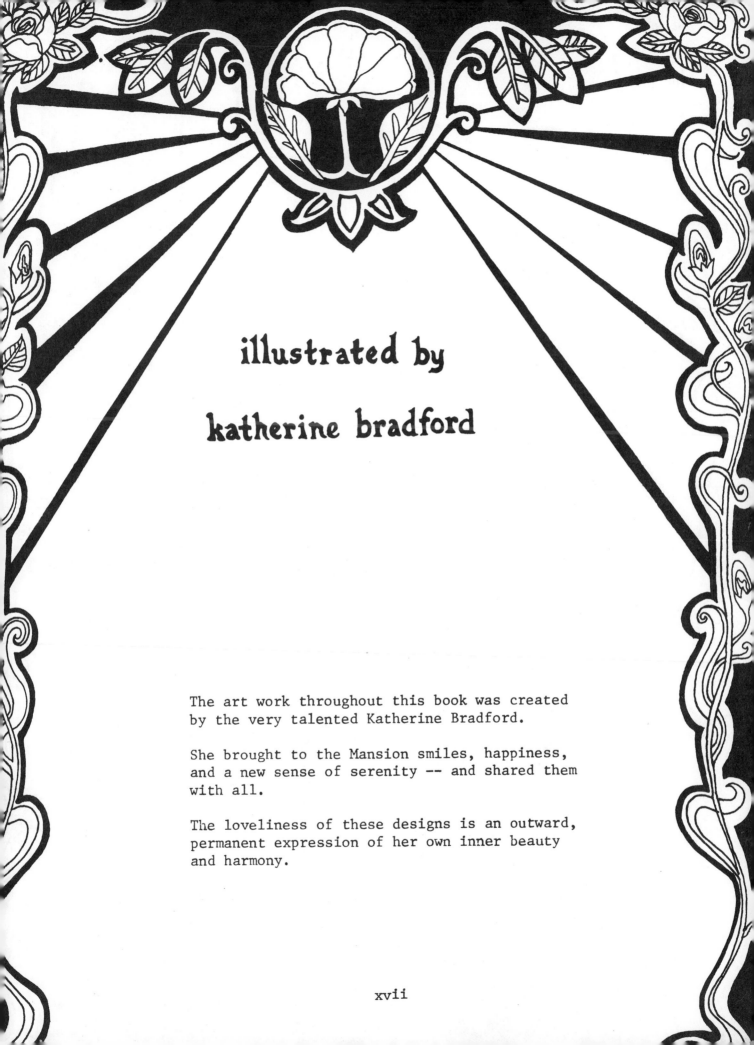

illustrated by

katherine bradford

The art work throughout this book was created
by the very talented Katherine Bradford.

She brought to the Mansion smiles, happiness,
and a new sense of serenity -- and shared them
with all.

The loveliness of these designs is an outward,
permanent expression of her own inner beauty
and harmony.

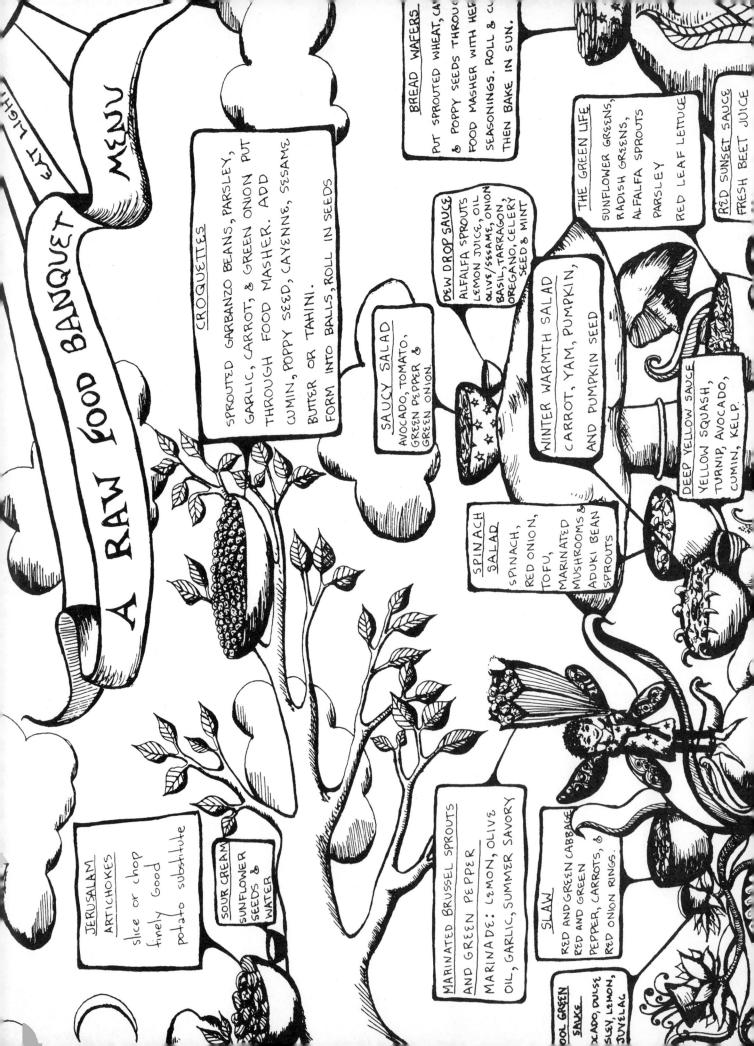

BASICS

TRANSITION DIET

The purpose of the transition diet -- from that of meat, processed foods, sugar, white flour products, etc., to a total living foods diet of vegetables, fruit, sprouts, fermented nuts, and seeds -- is to allow the body to gradually cleanse accumulated waste materials at a slower pace until the whole diet is one of living foods. Even while on the transition diet, attempt to incorporate as many green sprout salads and fruit meals as you comfortably can in order to speed up detoxification and to allow the body and mind to accustom themselves to this new diet.

The <u>first phase</u> in the transition diet is to eliminate drugs, medicines, and other chemicals; meat, tobacco, alcohol, white sugar, white flour, salt, and coffee -- all processed "foods." This may be a radical change for some people, as these "foods" have become deeply ingrained habits and dependencies. One way to approach this change is to "decrease and substitute." If you eat meat every day, for example, decrease it to two or three times a week, and substitute fish and fowl in its place. If you drink or smoke each day, cut it to every other day, then every third or fourth day. Substitute clearer thinking and deep, clean breathing exercises in their stead. You aren't giving anything up -- you are really choosing something better.

In the meantime, use as many live foods as possible as substitutes for the refined and processed foods. Use unfiltered honey and dates instead of sugar; whole grains instead of white flour; raw milk rennetless cheese instead of processed cheese; raw milk instead of homogenized milk; fresh fruits and vegetables instead of canned, frozen or packaged food. You'll notice a taste change, and in a short time your taste buds and mind will automatically choose nutritious foods.

The <u>second phase</u> in transition is the elimination of mucus-forming foods such as dairy products: milk, butter, cheese, eggs, yoghurt, etc. Begin to substitute seed milk cheese and seed yoghurt. While in this phase, try fasting on juices one day a week or more to expedite toxin elimination.

The <u>third phase</u> in transition is the elimination of all cooked foods from the diet. This includes grains, cooked fruits or vegetables, granola, crackers, all cooked legumes, bread, etc. The ultimate diet is that of fresh raw fruit and vegetables, sprouts, and fermented nuts and seeds. This transition may take months for some, perhaps only weeks or days for you. It's your decision.

Some additional transitional diet data:

1. Have three juice meals a day to nourish the body. Include a salad with each drink.
2. Clean out the colon with enemas and wheatgrass implants once or twice a day.
3. If you cook or steam vegetables, cook as little as possible, on the lowest heat possible, to retain the maximum amount of nutrients.
4. Eat the living foods before the cooked foods.
5. Try not to drink liquids for an hour after mealtimes.
6. Chew your food very, very well.
7. Find out more about food combining and digestion and begin using only the foods that are easily digested.

THE COMPLETE MEAL SALAD

Certain aspects of nutrition may be considered within the realm of science. An analysis of Dr. Wigmore's Complete Meal Salad has been prepared by Dr. Harvey C. Lisle, a graduate in Chemical Engineering from the University of Ohio, with fifteen years' industrial experience in food testing laboratories, including both animal and human foods. Over the years, he observed the natural superiority of health in families raised on natural foods and became convinced that the health enrichment of Americans lies in their abandoning highly refined and processed foods and returning to naturally produced foods.

The ingredients required in a complete meal are protein, carbohydrates, minerals, vitamins, and enzymes in sufficient quantity and quality to furnish adequate energy (or calories), and elements needed for growth (or maintenance). A meal prepared from raw garden produce, sprouts, and seeds will assuredly be rich in vitamins, minerals, and enzymes. By added a little dulse or kelp to the meal, flavor is enhanced and minerals are enriched beyond any doubt of adequacy. Such a meal provides a wide range of vitamins, minerals, and enzymes.

Animal protein has to be broken down into simple amino acids before it can be reconstructed into human protein. In meat eaters, putrefactive bacteria predominate, and most of the meat rots in the lengthy human intestines, placing an excessive strain on the liver, which is not equipped to eliminate large quantities of uric acid and other toxic by-products of meat eating. These toxins are often absorbed into the tissue of the organism.

In plant life, much of the protein is already in a predigested state; this is especially true of sprouts and indoor greens in which most of the protein is in the form of simple amino acids. Furthermore, the protein in plants has the advantage of being free from nucleo-proteins and therefore does not lead to the formation of uric acid in the system and does not encourage gout or rheumatism.

New scientific findings indicate the amount of protein required can vary from 20 to 50 grams for each individual, depending on weight, sex, climate, and type of work. Dr. M. Hindhede, Director of the Hindhede Laboratory for Nutritional Research established by the Danish Government, shows the definite relationshp between high protein diets and acidosis and disease. It is a scientifically demonstrated fact, for example, that dairy cows which are fed heavily on proteins are short-lived and subject to many disorders of the kidneys and bowels not found in cows permitted to graze and eat in a more normal manner.

It has been dramatically pointed out that a low protein diet in animals and humans yields an increased resistance to disease, and builds an immunity against cancer and that it is nearly impossible to graft cancer cells onto species fed on a low protein diet.

Protein is constructed of 22 building blocks called amino acids, of which eight have been found essential in the food requirements of people. From these eight, we can synthesize the others we require. All eight of these essential amino acids must be present together in the "complete meal" as they complement each other's qualities. If one of the eight is missing, then the remaining amino acids cannot be utilized and fail to provide what they were designed to.

The "Complete Meal Salad" contains full proteins in quantity and quality. A study of Table I will reveal the individual items which contain all eight of the essential amino acids. The sunflower seeds are especially excellent in this regard. Table II gives the necessary data from which the proteins and calories of Table III are calculated. Total protein for this one meal is 15 grams. Assuming the same amount of protein will be ingested during the other two meals of the day, the total protein intake will come to 45 grams.

Protein is very sensitive to heat. Heat causes irreversible changes in protein, changes that downgrade the protein. Most Americans now cook their food, whether meat or vegetable, which could account for the fact that most nutritionists recommend approximately 70 grams of protein per day for the average person, whereas raw food proponents recommend only about half that amount. Uncooked food can provide more usable proteins.

Table I — Based on 100 grams edible portions. Figures in milligrams.

	Isoleucine	Leucine	Lysine	Methionine	Phyenylanine	Tryptophane	Theonine	Valine
Avocado	--	--	120	19	--	23	--	--
Cucumber	9	13	13	3	7	2	8	10
Summer Squash	213	346	258	42	182	27	118	224
Greens	161	165	147	29	108	26	106	129
Sunflower Seeds	1320	1824	912	456	1272	360	936	1416
TOTAL	1703	2348	1450	549	1569	438	1168	1779

Table II

	% Protein	Calories per 100 grams
Avocado	2.1	245
Mung Bean Sprouts	3.8	23
Cucumber	0.6	12
Summer Squash	0.6	16
Leafy Greens	2.3	20
Sunflower Seeds	24.0	375
Coconut Oil	0	900
Tomato/Red Pepper	1.0	20

4

Table III.

	Portion	Weight (in grams)	Protein (in grams)	Calories
Avocado	1 quarter	50	1.0	122
Cucumber	7 slices	50	0.3	6
Mung Sprouts	1 cup	140	5.6	33.6
Summer Squash	1/2 cup	50	0.3	8
Sunflower Seeds	2 T	25	6.0	94
Leafy Greens	1/2 cup	25	0.6	5
Coconut Oil	1/8 cup	30	0.0	270
Dulse or Kelp	Few bits	10	0.0	0
Tomato/Red Pepper	2 slices	20	0.2	4
TOTAL		400	14.0	542.6

The average American eats too much food and takes in too many empty calories, energy units without vitamins and minerals. Our "complete meal salad" contains 543 calories -- vitamin, mineral and enzyme-packed calories. If the other two meals of the day contain the same number of calories, total caloric intake will total 1600.

Eating the highly processed foods of today negates the instinctive knowledge of how much and what to eat. Assuming that the person who partakes of the complete meal salad is on somewhat of a natural food regime, he or she will instinctively know whether the meal is satisfying, is too much or is not enough. With good judgment and regained instinct, the individual may take the complete meal salad and adjust it to his or her own personal requirements. It will maintain good health in body, mind, and spirit.

COMPLETE MEAL SALAD FOR TWO

1 C mung sprouts
1 C alfalfa sprouts
1 C summer squash, grated
1 C mixed greens
1 half avocado, sliced
1/4 cucumber, sliced
4 slices tomato
4 slices red pepper
2 T sunflower seeds
2 T coconut oil
1 t kelp

Mix all. For greens, use buckwheat lettuce, sunflower greens, beet greens, spinach, romaine lettuce, or any dark green. See page 86 for additional recipes.

FERMENTED FOODS

As well as raw fruits and vegetables, fermented foods are also eaten at the Institute, the most popular being rejuvelac, sauerkraut, and fermented seed dishes. These foods are included in the diet for an important reason -- they are extremely rich in enzymes, predigested protein, and lactobacillus bacteria.

In a healthy person, the enzymes are manufactured by the body. It is thought that aging occurs because the body loses the ability to synthesize new enzymes. The researchers are now convinced that diseases are traceable to missing enzymes.

Food that is fermented is filled with enzymes. People known for longevity -- the Hunzas, the Georgians -- use much fermented food. In Georgia, Russia, people eat yoghurt, sour bread, sour milk, soured vegetables. They also eat naturally made sauerkraut and sour pickles. These people seldom have digestion problems.

Dr. Kuhl, a German researcher, has this to say regarding fermented foods:

> The natural lactic acid and fermentive enzymes which are produced during the fermentation process have a beneficial effect on the metabolism and a curative effect on disease. Lactic acid destroys harmful intestinal bacteria and contributes to the better digestion and assimilation of the nutrients. Fermented foods can be considered predigested foods: they are easily digested and assimilated even by persons with weak digestive organs. Fermented foods improve the intestinal tract and provide a proper environment for the body's own vitamin production within the intestines. They also help a person with constipation problems.

REJUVELAC -- THE ENZYME DRINK

> Rejuvelac is rich in proteins, carbohydrates, dextrines, phosphates, saccharines, lactobacilli, saccharamyces, and aspergillus oryzae. Amylases are derived from aspergillus oryzae and they have the faculty of breaking down large molecules of glucose, starch, and glycogens. This is the reason rejuvelac is an aid to your digestion.
>
> (Dr. Harvey C. Lisle, Food Chemist)

Rejuvelac, the "water" of the Institute, puts into your body the enzymes cooked food doesn't. Enzymes help friendly bacteria such as lactobacillus bifidus to grow. Lactobacillus in turn gives off lactic acid, a natural astringent, which helps your large intestine maintain its natural, healthy, vitamin-producing environment. This leads to a clean colon where sludge does not collect on colon walls, and where harmful, disease-producing bacteria are unable to survive.

REJUVELAC

Rejuvelac is a pre-digested food -- the proteins are broken down into amino acids, the carbohydrates into simple sugars (dextrines and saccharines). These nutrients are readily assimilated by your body with little expenditure of energy. Rejuvelac is extremely rich in eight of the B vitamins, as well as Vitamin E and K.

Rejuvelac is also used as a "starter" in the production of other fermented dishes, particularly the protein (nut and seed) sauces, cheeses, and loaves. Drink glasses of it between meals to flush the system out, and help cleanse the intestinal tract.

TO MAKE REJUVELAC:

> (For approximately 3 cups)
> You will need: 1 C wheat berries (organic soft white pastry wheat)
> 3 C spring or filtered water
> a container -- a glass jar with a wide mouth

1. Wash seed by rinsing well (in tap water), and scrubbing seeds with hands to remove any outer residue. Allow dead seeds to float to top of container -- skim them off and discard -- they will not promote fermentation.
2. Soak the wheat berries the first time for 48 hours. (The seed is becoming porous.) Place a small, neat bundle of freshly cut wheatgrass on top of water for further filtering. Remove each day before pouring rejuvelac off; replace.
3. After 48 hours, pour off your rejuvelac. Use that for the day. It needn't be refrigerated, but will keep several days if it is.
4. Pour another 2 cups of spring or filtered water into the jar. Allow water to ferment only 24 hours before pouring off.
5. Repeat 24 hour cycles for 3 days, so wheat berries are soaked a total of 3 times.

A dark quiet place is ideal for setting your jars. The temperature of the fermenting environment is important. Warmer temperatures will decrease fermenting times. In the summer, try soaking the seed 36 hours to start, and 16 hours instead of 24. Ferment the rejuvelac to your taste -- until tart, not sour.

You can experiment and use any hulled seed — try different varieties of wheat, or millet, oats, rice, barley, rye, buckwheat, etc. At all times, use only organic seed. For uses of spent seed, see Essene bread, and living bread recipes, pages 138 and 140.

> Basic recipe: 1 part organic spring wheat (soft pastry wheat)
> 2 parts spring water
> Fermenting time remains the same for all quantities.

SAUERKRAUT

Sauerkraut is a vitamin-producing food which has been a boon to us for centuries, regulating our digestive processes, overcoming vitamin and mineral deficiencies, stimulating our bodies to a longer life, and above all, providing us with all the benefits of green and leafy vegetables at all times of the year -- as well as adding to our diet substances which other vegetables lack.

Sauerkraut supplies food lime and iron -- bone and blood builders -- and other vitamins and essential minerals. The pleasant, sour taste has a stimulating effe and helps the appetite. Elemental and frequent cases of intestinal catarrh are relieved by sauerkraut juice soup.

There are a great number of persons who cannot digest cabbage easily and who are troubled by "gas." We suggest that they try sauerkraut. In many cases, sauerkra is easier to digest and causes no aftereffect. Each person must judge for him/ herself whether cabbage or sauerkraut is the food which agrees best with his or her digestive system.

In plants and fruits provided us by Nature are a great abundance of all the vital ingredients needed to replenish our bodies. The surface of the earth was once covered with vegetation. There was a great variety of self-seeding plants which drew sustenance from the earth and multiplied with great vigor. Although we knew nothing about vitamins and calories in those early times, we managed to survive because our everyday diets included necessary amounts of both. The Divine Force directed ancient inhabitants of this earth to select from the abundance of wild plants precisely those foods which contain what is necessary for life and health -- the green, leafy plants, such as cabbage, which guarantee a long and disease-free life.

It was left to our ingenuity to select from among those many and varied plants those which could be stored without spoilage, in order to provide ourselves with essential foods during the non-productive seasons of the year. Widely used was sauerkraut, the fermented dish made from cabbage. Even today, sauerkraut means health to many peoples of the world, as well as an extraordinary sense of well-being, an economical and satisfying food, an easily-digested vegetable which combines in a most savory manner with other foods, and also -- as indicated by the experience of centuries -- a food which seems to prolong life.

For people of earlier times, sauerkraut was a tremendous discovery. They knew instinctively that life was jeopardized unless at least one green-leafed plant was included in their diet. In northern regions of the world, where winter came early and stayed late and the bare earth was covered for months with a thick blanket of snow, sauerkraut meant life for man until spring came again and the soil could produce foods to supply his needs. Sauerkraut was a substitute for fruits which could not be grown or stored in wintertime. It was a substitute for the many plants grown in the garden or gathered in the fields which could not be stored in winter without spoiling.

Cabbage is truly a remarkable plant. There is no other vegetable to compare with it. It is easy to cultivate and grows almost anyplace where the summer is humid and fairly long. It is truly Nature's gift to mankind.

FERMENTED SEED DISHES

Many preparations fall under the heading "Seed Dishes." These include nut or seed loaf, fermented protein sauce, seed yoghurt or seed cheese, seed cream, seed sauce, nut cheese, fermented nut or seed sauce, protein loaf.

Protein is a very concentrated food, more taxing to your digestive organs than any other raw food. By "predigesting" your proteins through fermentation, you give your body these required elements in a readily assimilable form. The proteins are broken into their amino acid components, easily absorbed, and do not have time to decompose. At the same time, you are taking in through the fermentation process enzymes to aid your digestion further.

To make -- follow the chart. Mix ingredients to the proper consistency, adding ground seed or rejuvelac as necessary. Add finely chopped vegetables (the more finely chopped, the more the individual flavors will spread through the dish). When you add the vegetables before fermenting, the vegetables will break down slightly and further yield their flavors. Or you can add them later, just before serving. See specific recipes for exact amounts of vegetables and spices, remembering that you are the creator; your intuition and fine sense will tell you far better than any recipe what your individual creation needs for completion.

Allow fermentation to occur at room temperature. The exact time of fermentation depends upon the temperature -- in summer, less time is needed. When the cheeses, yoghurts, and sauces ferment, the airier fermentation will take place on top, the heavier liquids (whey) will settle to the bottom, so mix your preparation once or twice for a smoother consistency. The seed firms up slightly during fermentation and tastes becomes stronger. Always use organic seed. Grind to a fine meal with a hand grain mill, or an electric nut/seed/coffee grinder.

Experiment with different nuts and seeds for different tastes. Sesame has a sharp taste, almonds are sweeter, and sunflower seeds give a blander flavor. Cashews are very rich, and peanuts very hard to digest.

If you use spring water instead of rejuvelac, triple the fermentation time. You can alter the fermentation time for any recipe. The less fermenting, the less tart the taste will be. All fermented dishes will keep refrigerated at least 3 to 5 days. Even though predigested, protein is still a concentrated food, so enjoy a few ounces at a time!

	SAUCE	CHEESE	LOAF
GROUND SEED	1 cup	2 cups	2 cups
REJUVELAC	2 cups	2 cups	1/3 cup
MIX TO CONSISTENCY OF	pancake batter	thick cottage cheese	thick dough
FERMENTING TIME	4 - 8 hours	12 - 24 hours	24 - 28 hours
CONTAINER	Put in bowl, cover w. plate	Put in bowl, cover w. plate	Form a loaf, cover w. cloth
YIELD	2 cups sauce	2 cups cheese	1 small loaf

BASIC SEED SAUCE

1/2 C sunflower seed	1/4 C sesame seed
1/4 C almond seed	1 C rejuvelac

Grind seed to fine meal. Blend with rejuvelac to a pancake batter consistency. Put in bowl, cover with a plate. Allow to ferment, at room temperature, 4 - 8 hours. Stir before serving.

If you desire a thicker sauce, add in a bit more meal, using the blender for greater smoothness. If sauce tastes a bit tart (over-fermented), put in a few drops of tamari or a teaspoon of minced onion to neutralize the taste.

Try making this sauce with just one type of seed; experiment with different types of seed. See the chapter on dressings for more seed sauce variations.

BASIC SEED CHEESE

1 C sunflower seed, ground	2 C rejuvelac	1 T kelp
1 C almond seed, ground		2 T tamari

Blend all. Allow to ferment 12 - 24 hours in covered bowl. Put bowl in warm place -- over a radiator or in a sunny window. Mix once or twice, gently, during fermentation.

BASIC SEED LOAF

1 C sunflower seed	1/2 C sesame seed	1 T kelp
1/2 C almond seed	1/3 C rejuvelac	1 T tamari

Grind seed. Mix all into a thick dough, adding rejuvelac as necessary. Pat into a loaf, cover with a white cloth and allow to set approximately 30 hours. Taste your loaf as it ferments. The longer it sets, the stronger the flavors will become.

To serve both the loaf and the cheese, roll into individual balls or patties, and place in a salad. Or stuff pepper slices with the mixture; hollow out cherry tomatoes and stuff those. Serve as hors d'oeuvres, or as a decorative salad addition. The loaf can also be left whole, decorated, and sliced when served. For more seed preparation ideas, see pages 152-153.

SEED LOAF WITH VEGETABLES

1 C almond seed	4 T pepper, minced	4 T minced mushrooms
1/2 C sunflower seed	4 T parsley, minced	2 T tamari
1/2 C sesame seed	4 T celery, minced	1 T kelp
1/3 C rejuvelac	4 T onions, minced	1 T sweet basil

Mix all, form into loaf, and ferment. For a cheese, alter rejuvelac and fermentation.

SPROUTS

From a tiny seed comes a sprout which is bursting with a life force that contains the necessary elements the body needs for normal growth and health. Since it is practically impossible to get organically grown fresh food in most places, this simple way to produce nourishment, which is superior to anything else cost-wise, is well worth learning.

Sprouting can be great fun and a real adventure. It is a wise, health giving hobby that will pay for itself many times over. Sprouts will grow in any climate, require no soil or sunshine, and cause no waste in preparation. For five cents it is possible to raise enough mung bean sprouts for a most nutritious meal. Sprouts are full of vitamins, minerals and quantities of protein in their purest form, and are readily digested with the help of the many enzymes they contain. Sprouts are an excellent source of Vitamins A, B-complex, C, D, E, G, K, and even U, and the minerals such as calcium, magnesium, phosphorous, chlorine, potassium, sodium, and silicon. They are all in natural forms which the body can readily assimilate.

Why sprout? Here are a few more reasons.

1. Sprouting is a quick, easy and inexpensive way to have a steady supply of fresh greens throughout the year.
2. The nutrients of grains, seeds, and legumes increase many times over when they are sprouted. Vitamins such as C, B, and E show gains of 10-20% when sprouted.
3. Sprouting allows you to raise your own indoor garden -- any time, any place, anywhere.
4. Sprouts can be used in thousands of ways. See recipes that follow for inspirations.
5. Sprouted grains and legumes supply all eight essential amino acids.
6. Many of the proteins in sprouts are pre-digested or broken down into their constituent amino acids, making them easily absorbable by the body, even for those with weak digestive organs.
7. The high level of simple sugars in sprouts puts them in the category of quick energy foods.
8. Sprouts are packed with enzymes -- the complex catalysts which initiate and control almost every chemical reaction taking place in a human.
9. Sprouts are a stable food -- they retain their enhanced nutritive values even after dehydration or freezing.

HOW TO SPROUT

Almost any seed, grain or legume can be sprouted, although some are tastier than others. Try them all! Seeds can be found in most natural foods stores. Be sure that the seeds or grains have not been chemically treated. If they have been, the germination rate will drop. Broken and chipped seeds also will not sprout. One ounce of dry seed equals about one cup of mature sprouts.

EQUIPMENT

A wide-mouth jar, such as a mason jar
Cheesecloth or wire mesh to cover the mouth, and
A rubber band or string to secure the mesh
The seeds or beans you wish to sprout. Make sure the jar has enough room for seeds to expand at least 8 times their present size. For example, 3 tablespoons of alfalfa will fill a quart jar.

SOAKING

Put seeds in jar and cover with mesh or cheesecloth, secure with rubber band. Wash seed by rinsing several times. Then fill up jar about halfway with lukewarm, preferably spring, water. See chart for exact soaking times. Set jar in a dark warm cupboard or shelf.

DRAINING

After the seeds have been soaked, drain off the water; save for soup stock. Rinse sprouts with fresh water, pour off. Now let sprouts rest by tilting jar upside down, at a 45⁰ angle, making sure that the mesh opening allows air in and isn't completely covered up by sprouts. A dish rack is useful for this.

RINSING

Rinse and drain well 2 or 3 times a day for 3 to 5 days. Use lukewarm water. Be sure the sprouts are sufficiently and continually drained as too much water and too little air will lead to molding and spoilage. Rinsing is basically making sure sprouts are kept moist. See chart for more exact timing.

That's all there is to it! Alfalfa sprouts need to be set in the sun after 5 days so they can start to manufacture chlorophyll. Remember that the time it takes for sprouts to mature will vary -- it depends on the temperature and humidity. Shorten soaking times for hotter, more humid weather, and rinse the sprouts more frequently to keep them cool. Sprouts are most tender when young, and they refrigerate well. They will keep for several days.

SPROUT CHART

SEED	SOAK (hours)	RINSE (times a day)	READY IN (days)
ADUKI	8-12	3	3-5
ALFALFA	5-8	2-3	5-6
CHICK PEAS (Garbanzo Beans)	8-15	4	3-4
CORN	8-15	3	2-3
FAVA BEANS*	8-12	3	3-4
FENUGREEK	6-8	3	3-4
LENTILS	8-12	3	2-3
MILLET	5-8	3	3-4
MUNG	8-12	4	5-6
OATS	5-8	2	3-4
PEAS	8-15	2	3-5
RADISH	5-8	2	3-5
RED CLOVER	5-8	4	5-7
RYE	8-12	3	2-3
SOYBEANS	15-24	4	3-4
SUNFLOWER SEEDS	8	2	24 hours
WHEAT	8-15	2	2-3

*and any bean: black, white, haricot, kidney, lima, navy, pinto, red, etc.
Grain sprouts are ready when the root is the length of the seed.

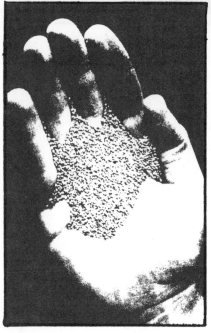

Seed or Grain
(Measured)

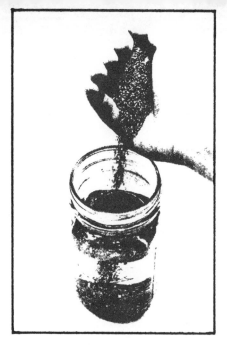

Place in water to soak

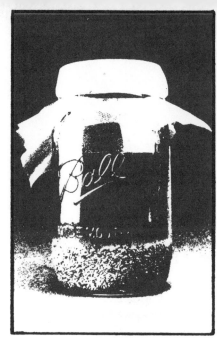

Soak according to type
of seed

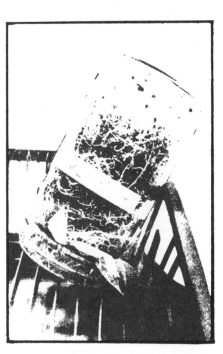

Place at 45° angle
to sprout

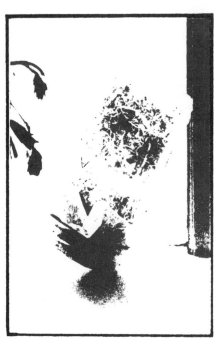

Place in window to
develop chlorophyll

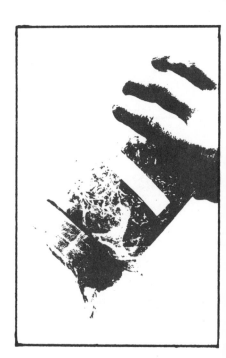

Rinse every 12 hours

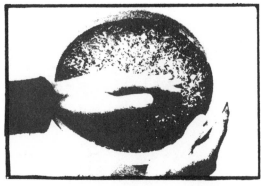

Remove hulls by placing
sprouts in water

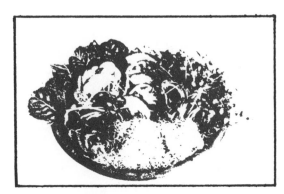

Use in your favorite
salad recipe

14

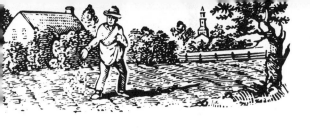
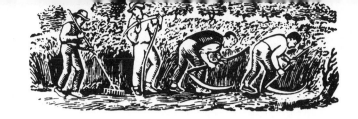

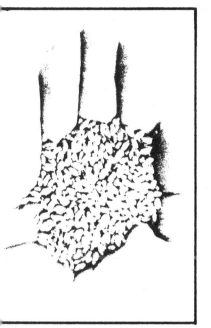

Whole Wheat Berries
(Measured)

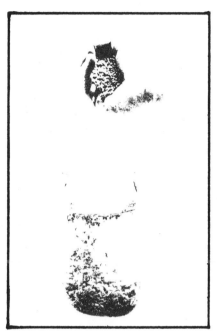

Place in Water & Soak

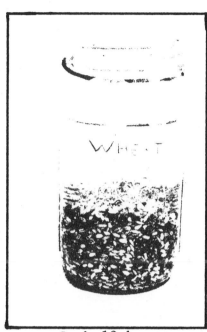

Soak 12 hours

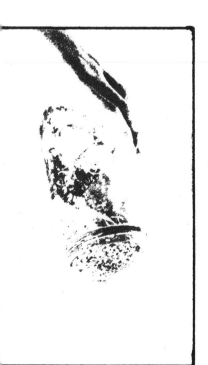

cain & Sprout 12 hours

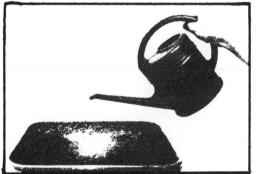

Spread soil 1-1/2"
thick, moisten

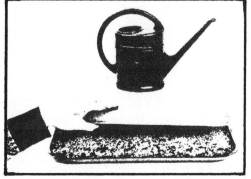

spread wheat evenly
over tray & cover

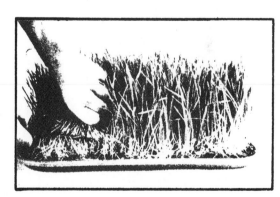

uncover water daily & harvest
close to roots on day 7

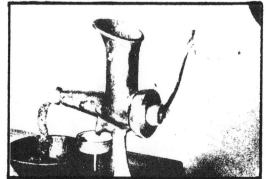

juice or chew grass

WHY GREENS?

Dr. E. H. Earp-Thomas, a researcher in the field of natural foods, maintains that grass, grown organically, provides one of the most powerful types of food grown by Mother Nature. All life on this planet is maintained primarily by the sun. Plants know how to capture the solar energy and mix it with the elements of air and water. Sun energy, air, and water are reinforced with minerals from the earth, absorbed through the roots of the plant, and this arrangement enables the human bloodstream to receive the elements so necessary for cleansing and building. In fact, Dr. Wilstatter of the University of Pennsylvania found that the elements making up the chlorophyll in plants are approximately the same elements from which red blood cells are constructed. Therefore, he pronounced chlorophyll the ideal food medicine.

Chlorophyll cleanses, heals, and builds the body cells. It banishes anemic conditions quickly, reduces blood pressure, and aids the heart action. It frees clogged arteries, smoothes out arthritic conditions, and improves the peristalsis (the contractions that occur along the digestive track, moving the food along in the digestive process). As a result of a diet rich in chlorophyll, the health is improved and a happier mental outlook is experienced.

COMPOSTING

Before getting into growing indoor greens, it is important to discuss soil and composting. The soil is where the nutrients come from. Fertile soil is no accident, and must be worked on. Organic gardening improves soil by increasing its organic content.

Composting is nature's way of building new soil through the decomposition of natural plant materials. Composting costs nothing and takes little effort. All sorts of organic wastes can be used -- table scraps, leaves, grass clippings, weeds, etc. Compost is more than fertilizer; it is the process of continuing life.

A true gardener appreciates the valuable assistance of earthworms since they will aerate the soil and enrich the mineral content. The earthworm actually eats and digests the soil. Its excrement is richer in minerals than the ingested soil. Chemical fertilizers and sprays are fatal to earthworms. Obtain earthworms from natural country soil, or from a bait and tackle fishing store. Ask for red wigglers.

If you do not have a shed or an area in the basement you can section off and use for decomposing soil, you will need one or more large trash cans, whatever space permits. Obtain the best soil you can find, preferably soil which has not been sterilized or chemically treated. If you are unable to obtain earth from the country, or a backyard, use the sterilized earth sold in stores. The earthworms and decomposing table scraps will add life to it.

COMPOSTING CAN

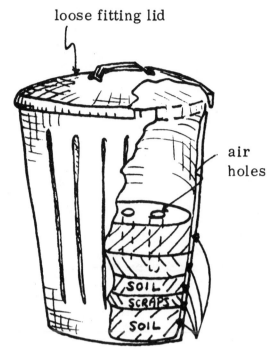

loose fitting lid

air holes

layered soil with worms and scraps

1. Fill the bottom of your trash can with soil, about 2 to 3 inches deep, and add 3 or 4 earthworms.

2. On top of this layer, place fruit and vegetable scraps. Cover them with an inch or two of soil. Harvest soil (the mats from cut indoor greens) may be added on top of this.

3. Each day, follow the same procedure, covering scraps with soil and greens.

4. Three to four times a week, aerate the soil by punching deep holes into it with a broomstick or mop handle.

5. For further ventilation, make sure the top of the can fits loosely and is open enough for air to get in and circulate.

6. When filled, the soil inside the can will be ready to use in 6 to 8 weeks.

GREENS YOU CAN GROW INDOORS

There are basically two types of greens one can grow indoors -- those with soil and those without. The most practical greens to grow with soil are wheatgrass, buckwheat lettuce, and sunflower greens, all of which take only seven days to grow. Buckwheat lettuce and sunflower greens may be used in salads or for juicing. The juiced wheatgrass is especially important to have as its chlorophyll is a powerful blood cleanser; the grass itself helps purify the air, and a handful of grass in drinking water or bath water helps neutralize the chemical content of the water.

The greens grown without soil are, of course, sprouts. The easiest to grow for obtaining chlorophyll are alfalfa and the clovers. These also take about seven days to grow, and may be used in salads or for juicing.

All greens should be grown from organically grown seed as these are the most nutritious. Sprays and fertilizers lodged in plant fibers or seed are poisonous to the human system. Seeds from sprayed plants do not grow or sprout well.

HOW TO PLANT

Obtain organic, unhulled sunflower seed and buckwheat seed, and organic hard red winter wheat. Pick out any damaged chipped or cracked seed. Buy baking trays

17

from a restaurant supply store, or use an available container -- pie plate, casserole dish, a cardboard box lined with plastic or foil. Cafeteria trays are convenient also.

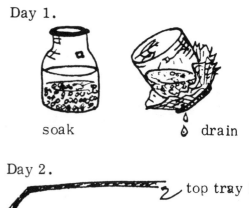

Day 1.

soak   drain

Soak the seed 8 - 15 hours. For best germination results, allow seed to drain 8 hours before planting.

Mix the earth you use with wet peat moss. This will assure good ventilation and drainage for developing roots. Spread the soil about one inch thick in your tray. Work the earth with your hands so it is loose and smooth. Form a trench along two sides.

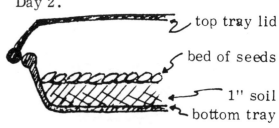

Day 2.

top tray lid
bed of seeds
1" soil
bottom tray

Now, wet the soil thoroughly, but not so much as to form pools of water, or to make mud.

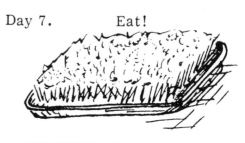

Day 7.   Eat!

Spread a layer of seed over the soil. Each seed should touch another on all sides, but should not have any others on top of it. In other words, all the seeds should have access to the soil, and form a thick carpet covering the earth.

GROWING INDOOR GREENS

Cover this layer of seed with 4 - 8 pieces of soaking wet newspaper (4 pieces in hot humid weather, up to 8 in colder, dryer weather). Finally, place a piece of plastic over that to prevent the newspapers from drying out. Allow plastic edges to drape over the tray, do not tuck underneath, as the seeds need air to grow. Instead of using paper and plastic, use another tray as a top cover.

Growth will make whatever top cover you use rise. On the fourth day, remove the sheets or tray, and save for later use. Water the greens (this will be their first drink). Place the tray in the sunlight, or where there is plenty of daylight. Be sure to water the greens daily (once in the morning is recommended) as there is not enough soil to retain moisture.

On the seventh day, the greens will be at their peak. The buckwheat and sunflower greens will be from 5 - 7" tall, the wheatgrass, about 7 or 8" tall. Cut all greens as close to the base as possible. This is where the majority of vitamins are stored.

If the soil is very rich, you might allow a second crop to come up; however, the second crop is never as thick as the first. Otherwise, remove the harvested mat from the tray and place it, face down, into your compost can and allow it to decompose.

ENTREES

GRAIN CRISPS

Variety of nourishment and the need for concentrated and valuable nutrients to take care of the immediate needs of unhealthy people is important. At Hippocrates Institute, we have added grain crisps to the standard diet to help furnish these needed nutrients. But, it is not advisable for cancer victims to eat such concentrated food.

Grain crisps are very simple to make. Grains used can be rice, millet, barley, oats, rye, and/or wheat. With the exception of rice, all are soaked for twelve hours; rice is soaked for twenty-four hours. Next, the grain should be sprouted another twelve hours. The sprouted grain is then blended with rejuvelac -- generally one cup of grain to one cup of rejuvelac.

As you blend, different flavors can be added. For a banana grain crisp, you would use two bananas to one cup of grain and one cup of rejuvelac. Blend together and pour on a drying sheet. For cinnamon grain crisp, add about two tablespoons of cinnamon to your paste. If you want a sweeter grain crisp, add some soaked dates, or you can add raisins. For an herb flavor, add an herb mixture, and for a vegetable grain crisp, you can add onions or any desired vegetable. Sea vegetables can also be used: dulse, kelp, or Irish moss, and they will provide needed minerals, as well as vitamins E, D, and A, and calcium and magnesium. Place mixture in dehydrator until crisp.

DRIED FOODS

A very helpful way to eat while traveling is to keep on hand dried foods. Bananas are good dried -- just cut them into thin pieces and put them in the dehydrator. They can be dried at the same time as the grain crisps. Another good snack is dried zucchini squash. It can be kept in a plastic bag and served as a fortification against the temptation to eat unhealthy foods while traveling.

Seasonings can also be dried: onions, parsley, scallions, and any herb which has been grown in your garden -- especially mint, if you are still taking mint tea. Any vegetables lying unused in your refrigerator can be sliced and put into the dehydrator at the same time as your grain crisps. For reasons of economy, be sure to utilize all the space the dehydrator offers; generally, there are about eight drying trays, and these can be filled up with an unlimited number of foods.

COCONUT OIL

We do not advocate the use of oil because it is denatured by processing. Therefore, we advocate avocado, seeds, and coconut, all of which are excellent replacements for denatured oil. When a recipe calls for oil, you can use oil which has been skimmed from blended coconut. The simple process is as follows:

1. With a screwdriver, bore a hole in the "mouth" of the coconut (i.e., the lower of the three soft spots). Drain the liquid and reserve it for a delicious drink.

2. Place coconut in a sturdy plastic bag and secure opening of bag. Then, with a hammer or other heavy instrument, smash the coconut into manageable pieces.

3. With a screwdriver or small kitchen knife, pry the meat of the coconut from the pieces of shell.

4. Pour some rejuvelac into your blender and start the machine. _Gradually_ add the pieces of coconut meat to the blender.

The coconut oil will rise to the top of the resultant mixture and this oil may be skimmed off and used whenever a dish calls for oil. It will keep in the refrigerator for two or three days. The blended coconut meat may be strained for milk, taken as cereal for breakfast, or used in pies or other dishes in which you would use nuts.

HEALTHY MEALS ON A SMALL BUDGET

We Americans are habituated to a schedule of three meals a day, plus snacks, and the state of our health suffers accordingly. What is being introduced to you here, however, is the ideal diet for bringing the whole family to a state of perfect health and well-being. It is a question of changing habits, and you are the best judge of the rate at which this can be done. While in a period of transition to living foods, it is best to allow your body to accept new food materials into the system, to incorporate new eating patterns so thoroughly that they will become lifetime habits, rather than being discarded as soon as weight is lost or physical problems overcome.

Following are some suggestions for the new eating habits you will develop:

Breakfast

The first meal of the day should be a light one. The digestive organs may not yet have awakened and may not be ready for the stimulation of heavy food. Also, a light morning meal is best if one wishes to have an alert mind. If you are used to a big meal in the morning, you can begin by reducing your intake, perhaps substituting a few pieces of fruit for your usual meal. As you do so, bear in mind the rules of food combining: acid and sour fruits should never be mixed with sweet fruits; sub-acid fruits blend fairly well with either of these categories; and melons should be eaten alone.

If you choose not to eat first thing in the morning, you can use the time otherwise spent at breakfast for meditation, exercise, work or study.

Drinking sprout and green juices is another satisfying way to give your body light nourishment at breakfast time. Eight to twelve ounces of rejuvelac can be drunk first thing in the morning or for breakfast and will provide a quick lift. It contains much vitamin E, more vitamin C than orange juice, and a large quantity of enzymes to aid the digestion. Also, a buttermilk can make an ideal breakfast: simply mix two tablespoons of fermented seed sauce (see below) mixed with a glass of rejuvelac.

Lunch

This is the meal at which the greatest amount of food should be taken, because it is at a time of day when the sun's rays are most direct and our digestive energies are at their highest. Ideally, you should rest five minutes before and after the noon meal. Eating is a sacred act and should not be indulged in without full appreciation of it as such. Otherwise, we will not get maximum benefit from and assimilation of the food which is needed for nourishment of our cells. Lunch should never be rushed or burdened with business problems or other concerns. If possible, it should be eaten in silence.

A complete meal salad with dressing may be taken at the midday meal. Again, food combining rules should be borne in mind: proteins and starches should never be eaten together if food is to be properly assimilated; each of these goes better with greens than with fruits. (Tomatoes, although a fruit, usually are well digested with protein dishes.) Remember that proteins include seeds (uncooked or fermented), sprouted seeds, nuts, legumes, and avocados. These are the protein forms recommended. Starches include potatoes, corn, chickpeas, carrots, and other sweet tubers. Grains or seeds should be sprouted when used for milk or cereal.

Fermented Seed Sauce Preparation

This is perhaps easiest carried out in the morning with the grinding or blending of sunflower seeds, sesame seeds or other seeds, and almonds. These should be ground down to a fine meal or blended, with the quantity depending on your own needs.

Add to the amount of seed meal an equal amount of rejuvelac and blend it in the blender. After the mixture is smooth and creamy, it should be set aside at room temperature (68° - 75°) to ferment for about 5 hours. It can be used at this point, or it can be refrigerated for several days. Be creative with your seed ferment mixtures. You may mix half sunflower and half sesame seeds, for instance, for a variation in taste. From the base you can make many different kinds of sauces.

Fermented Seed Cheese

Blend equal amounts of sesame seeds, sunflower seeds, and rejuvelac, and allow the mixture to ferment for about five hours at room temperature, then put the mixture in a sprouting bag and hang up to drain for several days.

To this "cheese" can be added finely chopped vegetables; celery, green or red pepper, parsley, or cucumber; and/or kelp or ground herbs. Any of these will add variety and enhance the flavor of your cheese. Even though the seeds in the cheese are fermented, it is not recommended that you eat the cheese alone. It is very rich in protein and if too much of it is eaten unaccompanied by other food, it could be mucus-forming. It is suggested, therefore, that you enjoy a helping of seed cheese with a green salad -- perhaps one which includes a variety of sprouts.

Seed Loaves

Loaves are made in much the same way as cheese, the difference being that spices and vegetables can be added to the seed meal and rejuvelac mixture before fermentation. Then all the ingredients are allowed to ferment about five hours. One pleasant surprise about these fermented loaves is that they keep well for quite a long time -- up to several weeks, if necessary. The loaf develops a stronger taste as it continues to ferment, but it will not become rancid. The mold which eventually grows on such dishes is a beneficial type, the same as mold on cheeses, and may certainly be eaten. However, like cheese, this loaf should be eaten in small quantities, along with a sprout salad or other vegetable meals.

Sauerkraut

Sauerkraut is another fermented food that is served at the Institute for lunch.
The following is my recipe for this delicious and healthful food. It obviously
makes a large quantity, and you may want to reduce the amounts used to suit your
needs.

Dr. Ann's Pink Sauerkraut

In advance --

Shred about 14 heads of cabbage -- half red, half green -- and set aside
about 10 of the outer leaves.

Mix in a bowl 5 level tablespoons each of kelp powder and dried juniper
berries (ground, except for a few to be thrown in whole).

Add about 6 ounces of wakame.

Then --

Put three inches of the shredded cabbage into a five-gallon pail or
other non-breakable container. Sprinkle over this a heaping tablespoon
of the kelp/berries mixture, and on top of that spread one cup of the
wakame mixture. Pound all of these with a pestle or other pounding instrument until the juices flow.

Repeat this procedure in three-inch layers until all the ingredients are used.

Cover with the 10 outer cabbage leaves.

Place a plate on top of leaves and a weight on top of the plate. Cover
the hole with a dish cloth.

Leave at room temperature for about seven days, depending on climate and
season. Before removing sauerkraut, skim residue from side of container.
Store in jars in your refrigerator until used. The sauerkraut will keep
about one month.

Dinner

Because the sun's rays are less intense and our own vital energies on the
decrease towards evening, the last meal of the day, if taken, should be
somewhat lighter than the noontime meal.

Again, salad consisting either of greens, sprouts, or fresh vegetables or
fruits in proper combination may be eaten. Because fruit is easily digested,
it would probably make an ideal evening meal. This is not recommended, however,
in the case of the diabetic or hypoglycemic. A vegetable juice or Green Drink
for the evening meal presents another delicious possibility for nourishment.

For your greens and uncooked soups, you can prepare an almost endless variety of palate-pleasing, nourishing seed or vegetable sauces and dressings. By experimenting with food in new ways, you will certainly create a variety of healthy menus that will become favorites with you. Here are a few healthy family dinner recipes that can serves as models.

I.   SAUCES

Avocado Sauce

Blend together 1 cup each of the following: celery, parsley, and scallions, with 1 cup of rejuvelac. Add 1 cup of any combination of the following: squash, carrots, spinach, beets, or cauliflower. Add one-half avocado and blend entire mixture until creamy.

Pumpkin Sauce

Slice and grate about 2 handfuls of pumpkin.

Chop: 2 celery stalks (with leaves)
       2 scallions
       ½ tomato
       ½ avocado
       1 bell pepper
       small quantity of beets

Blend cut-up pumpkin and vegetables with some rejuvelac until smooth.

Tomato Sauce

Blend some tomatoes with fresh basil and parsley and ½ avocado.

II. SOUPS

Carrot Soup

Grate 5 medium carrots
Blend with 1 celery stalk, 2 scallions, ½ avocado
Add a dash of tamari or kelp
May be thinned with rejuvelac

Cream of Tomato Soup

Blend 1 or 2 medium tomatoes with:
½ avocado
1 sprig parsley
2 fresh basil leaves, if available
½ medium cucumber
2 red peppers
1 stalk celery

Other Ideas for Soups and Sauces

Use leftover vegetables with rejuvelac or water to blend and avocado for
flavor.

III. COMPANY MEALS

Just to show the range of possibilities of your new eating style, invite
friends over to share this "Italian spaghetti" or this delicious vegetable
loaf.

"Italian Spaghetti"

Chop tomatoes, celery, bell pepper, garlic, onion, basil, oregano,
and marjoram.

Serve over long sprouts (stems only), from buckwheat greens.

Vegetable Loaf

½ cup oats, sprouted and ground
1 cup rejuvelac
1 t kelp
¼ t oregano
2 stalks celery, chopped fine
1 cup seed cheese (prepared ahead of time)
4 large carrots, ground
1 medium red onion, ground
1 medium green pepper, chopped fine

Soak oats for about 10 hours by placing in bowl and covering with water;
then sprout for 10 hours more and grind.
Wash and grind into small pieces 4 large carrots
Wash and cut into very small pieces green pepper, celery, and onion
Put seasonings and rejuvelac and cheese into blender and mix.
Mix all ingredients in large bowl until well blended.

IV. SNACKS

Normally, snacks should be avoided, but if you must snack, you might
have a Green Drink or rejuvelac, carrot or celery sticks, or a piece
of fruit.

When entertaining, have treats that offer nutritious benefits to your
guests as well as to yourself. The following are healthful and tasty, but
to be eaten sparingly: some of them evade the rules of good food combining,
and the fruit sugars may overstimulate the appetite without nourishing the
body.

Smoothie

Blend one avocado, 4 apples, and tablespoonful of honey.

Frozen Banana Ice Cream

Freeze several peeled bananas (other fruit can be substituted for bananas). Put through juicer or blender. The result will be amazingly like soft ice cream. You may wish to sprinkle carob powder over it.

Pear Pudding

Blend until smooth equal amounts of peeled pears and bananas. Serve with currants and cinnamon.

Pies

For a special occasion, a raw pie may be made with a crust of ground coconut or seeds and honey or dried fruit as a binder, and a blended fruit sauce as a filling.

Top with rounds of bananas and other fruit slices or berries.

Raw Confections

Candies and cookies may be made from ground or chopped raisins, dates, figs, nuts, or seeds. These may be rolled in shredded or ground coconut.

The variety of confections is bounded only by your imagination. Try combining different soaked (overnight) dried fruits with fresh fruits and nuts or seeds. Add powdered carob when a chocolate taste is desired.

A Word About Seasonings

The seasonings suggested for use in any of the preceding recipes (or in any you may create) are:

Herbal Seasonings: parsley, garlic, onion, dill, marjoram, thyme, tarragon, basil, nutmeg, rosemary.

Seaweeds: powdered kelp, used as salt and flavoring; wakame; nori; etc.

Tamari: a fermented soy sauce which should be used very sparingly, as it contains a considerable amount of salt.

No seasoning, not even those listed above, should ever be used to excess, only to enhance the flavor of the dish. Our taste buds should relish the delightful flavors of unadulterated salads and other uncooked foods. Over a period of time, excessive seasoning can cause digestive and kidney problems. Because of their stimulative effects, they also tend to cause overeating.

Think of seasonings in this way: they should complement, not replace, the full, natural flavors of foods.

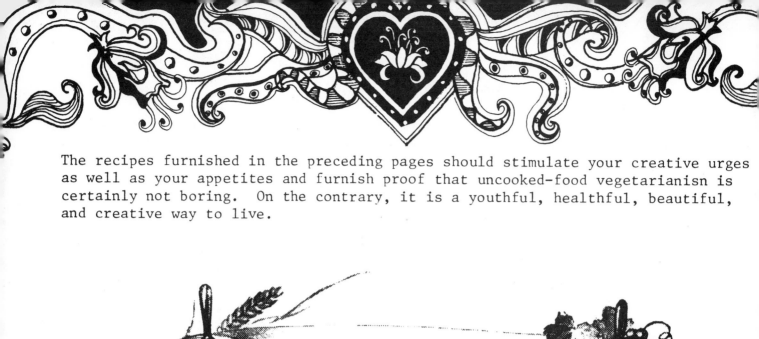

The recipes furnished in the preceding pages should stimulate your creative urges as well as your appetites and furnish proof that uncooked-food vegetarianisn is certainly not boring. On the contrary, it is a youthful, healthful, beautiful, and creative way to live.

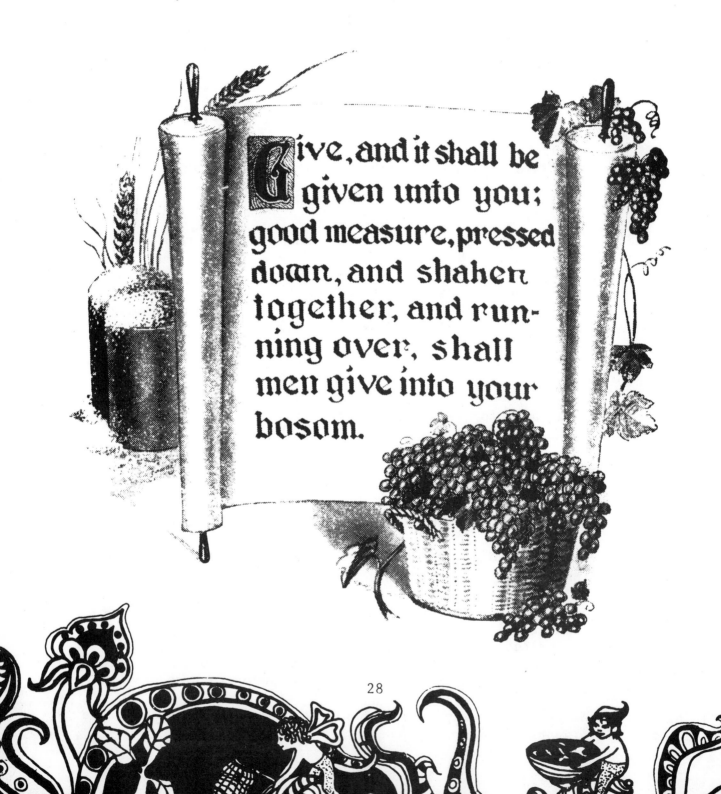

Give, and it shall be given unto you; good measure, pressed down, and shaken together, and running over, shall men give into your bosom.

CROQUETTES OF GARBANZOS AND CARROTS

1 C sprouted garbanzo beans (chickpeas), mashed
1/2 C parsley, finely chopped
1 cup carrots, homogenized
1/2 C green onion, minced
1 clove garlic, minced
Spices: Add to taste (1/4 t each, approximately) cumin, poppy
        seed, cayenne, sesame
1/2 C sunflower seeds, coarsley ground.

Combine all ingredients. Form into balls. Roll in coarsely ground
seeds, or serve as a salad on bed of sprouts. Makes 12 croquettes,
or a hearty salad for 2.

DECORATION IDEAS:

For a loaf or a cheese, sculpt into
imaginative shapes -- for the "Almost
Tuna Salad," form a fish; for the
chicken salad, a chicken. Pepper
slices can be used for mouths or
feet, and broccoli flowerettes for
eyes. Any preparation is made more
appetizing by being surrounded with
fresh greens or sprouts. On top of
the srpouts, put carrot and/or stuffed
celery sticks.

29

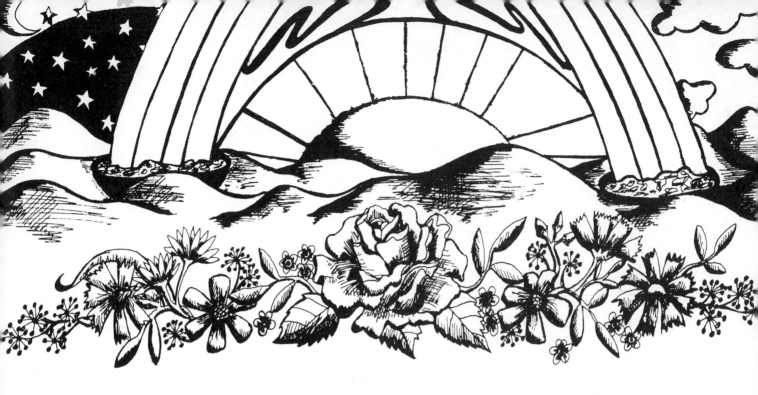

MOCK CHICKEN SALAD (Delicious!)

5 cups	lentil sprouts	1 T	Bronner's seasoning
2 cups	celery, minced	1 T	raw peanut butter
2 cups	fresh corn cut off cob	1 T	raw almond butter
1 cup	yellow pea sprouts	2 t	nutritional yeast
2	green onions with tops, minced	2 t	kelp

Put sprouts and fresh corn through homogenizer of Champion juicer or through another food grinder. Add all other ingredients; mix well. Serve raw. Make decorative patties, croquettes, or a loaf. Allow ingredients to sit for several hours in refrigerator before serving for flavors to increase. Serves 6 - 8.

TO DECORATE A LOAF:

Chop, sliver, or slice colorful vegetables: beets, watercress, red cabbage, tomatoes, celery, carrots, onions, etc. Place all in fanciful design over loaf or patties. Use contrasting colors to brighten the dish. Surround loaf by alternating sliced tomato with parsley or watercress sprigs. Or form concentric circles of red cabbage and dark greens. These are just a few ideas -- your variations will be unending!

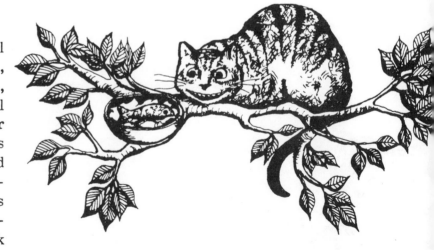

ALMOST TUNA SALAD

1 C alfalfa sprouts

1/4 C mung sprouts

1/4 C lentil sprouts

1/4 C chopped onion

1/4 C chopped parsley

1/2 C chopped celery

2-3 T seed sauce

2-3 T almond butter

1 T kelp (or more)

1 tomato

Combine celery, seed sauce, almond butter and kelp in blender until smooth. Add mung, lentils, onion, half of the parsley. Blend a few seconds until sprouts are just chopped. Stir blended mixture into alfalfa sprouts. Serve in tomato cups (halve the tomato, scoop out insides-- which can be added to a vegetable sauce), and garnish with the remainder of parsley. For 2 - 4.

QUICK TUNA

(A) 1 C celery, chopped

1 C sprouted wheat berries

(B) 1/2 C parsley, chopped

1/2 C sprouted chick peas

1/2 C sprouted lentils

2 T wheatgrass, finely cut

(C) 2-4 T tahini

2 T tamari

1 C alfalfa sprouts

1 C fenugreek sprouts

1 quart mixed sprouts:
alfalfa-mung-fenugreek

1/2 C Italian dressing

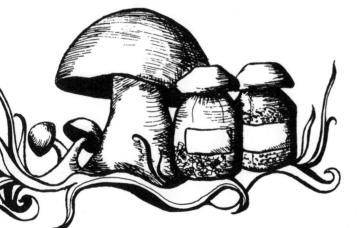

Homogenize column (A) and (B). Use a blender, hand juicer, a food grinder, potato masher, or a mortar and pestle. Now mash in column (C). Serve over the quart of mixed sprouts, covered with Italian dressing. Serves 6 - 8.

VEGETABLE SEED LOAF

1 C sunflower meal

1 C almond meal

1 C sesame meal

1/2 C rejuvelac

4-5 diced mushrooms

1/2 C parsley, diced

3 sticks celery, diced

1 clove garlic, diced

2 T tamari

1 t basil

1 t caraway seed

Mix all ingredients into a loaf, and ferment 24-48 hours. 6 - 8.

MEAT LOAF #1

1/2 C sunflower seed meal
1/2 C sesame meal
1/2 C chick pea meal (soak chick peas at least
6 T rejuvelac   24 hours before grinding)

1 1/2 C homogenized beet	1 T tamari
1 tomato, diced	1 T basil
1/2 red pepper, minced	1/2 t caraway seed, ground
1/4 C parsley, minced	1/2 t kelp

Ferment the seed meals 24-48 hours. Taste for flavor, and to see when the loaf is done. It will be slightly tart. Before serving, add finely chopped vegetables, beet and spices. The homogenized beet will give the loaf a pink color. Form into a loaf, place on a bed of greens. Or make individual servings with an ice cream scoop and place in separate bowls filled with greens and sprouts. For 4 - 6.

MEAT LOAF #2 (less fermentation)

1 C sunflower seed meal	1/2 C diced mushrooms
1 C pumpkin seed, ground	1/4 C minced parsley
1 C chick peas, ground	1 pepper, diced
1/2 C rejuvelac	

Blended Sauce
2 medium tomatoes
2 T basil
2 T tamari
1 T kelp
1 clove garlic, pressed

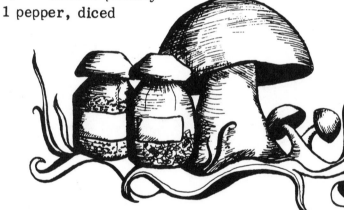

Start meal, rejuvelac and vegetables in the morning.
At dinner time, make sauce. Add in to the loaf about half; enough to give a looser texture. Form into a loaf. Put on a bed of greens and pour remaining sauce over all. For 6 - 8.

LENTIL LOAF

2 C soaked red lentils (24 hours)	1/2-1 C each: chopped tomatoes
1-2 carrots, well shredded	chopped celery
1 C sesame-sunflower seed meal	chopped bell pepper

Mix the seed meal with a few T's of the soak water -- form a doughy consistency. Mash lentils, blend vegetables. Mix all together. Shape into loaf.

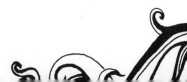

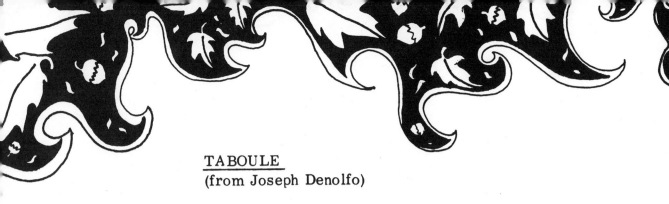

TABOULE
(from Joseph Denolfo)

1 C triticale (1/2 C wheat, 1/2 C rye or rice)
spring water

2-3 T each: chopped parsley
            chopped celery
            chopped onion
            chopped pepper

1 T coconut oil
1 T tamari
1/2 t each: paprika, basil,
                  cayenne pepper

Cover triticale with pure water, add in 1 more inch of water. Let soak 8-16 hours. Drain, save water for dressings and drinks. Allow seeds to sprout 2 days in loosely covered jar.

After they've sprouted, add chopped vegetables and spices. For 2 - 4. Try any other sprouted grains, and different vegetable additions.

Use taboule to stuff hollowed out peppers or large tomato halves for a festive entree.

'SPANISH' TABOULE

2 C taboule (use recipe above)
    2 medium tomatoes, chopped

1 t paprika
1/2 t cayenne pepper

Make taboule as above; blend the tomatoes and spices and pour the mixture over the sprouted grains. For 2.

JOSEPH'S DELIGHT

3 C sunflower seed cheese
1/2 C sauerkraut
1/2 avocado
3 T tamari
1 C each: alfalfa, fenugreek sprouts, or buckwheat, sunflower greens

Mix cheese, sauerkraut with dressing and tamari. Serve over sprouts and/or greens. For 4 - 6.

GUACAMOLE

1 medium tomato	1 medium tomato
1/2 red bell pepper	1/2 red bell pepper
1/2 small zucchini	1/2 small zucchini
2 T kelp	3 T minced onion
	1 t each paprika, basil, parsley
2 avocados	1/2 t cayenne pepper

Blend column 1 vegetables until smooth. Then mash in avocados, and add in well chopped or grated column 2 veggies for texture. Makes about 3 cups.

TOMATO CORONETS

2 large tomatoes	1 1/2 C alfalfa sprouts
1-2 T kelp	3 C guacamole

Slice the tomatoes, put on a platter. Sprinkle on kelp. Then add guacamole, and top with sprouts. Makes about 12 coronets.

Variation: Instead of a sliced tomato base, hollow out 3 or 4 smaller tomatoes. Add that pulp to the blended guacamole filling. Stuff tomato bases, and top with sprouts.

SPICY CHICK PEA SPROUTS

3 C sprouted chick peas	1/4 C minced onion
4-6 T coconut oil	1 T paprika
1/4 C parsley, minced	1 t herbal seasoning

Mash the chick peas in the oil -- use a potato masher, mortar and pestle, or whiz quickly in the blender. Add in all other ingredients. For 2 - 4.

Variations: Use different grain sprouts -- triticale, barley, wheat, oats.
Try 1/4 C of chopped mustard greens in place of the parsley and paprika.
Use this as a stuffing for peppers and tomatoes.

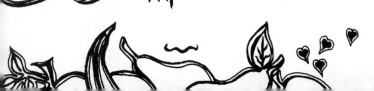

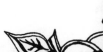

MUSHROOM LOAF

4 C chopped mushrooms
2 C chopped bell peppers

Sauce:
2 avocados
2 scallions
1/2 C rejuvelac
1/4 C sunflower seed sauce
pinch of oregano

Decorations:
1/2 C parsley, minced
1 large tomato, sliced

Blend sauce and pour over mushrooms and peppers. Oil a bowl and put mixture in. Pat down, and turn over onto a flat plate. Decorate with parsley and tomatoes. For 6 - 8.

NUT LOAF #1001

2 C homogenized carrot
1/2 small onion, finely chopped
1/4 C parsley, finely chopped

1/2 C ground almonds
1/2 C ground cashews
2 T coconut oil
2 T vegetable seasoning

Mix ingredients together. Shape into loaf and decorate. Serve over individual plates of greens. For 2 - 4.

CARROT SALAD WITH CREAMED ALMOND CHEESE

2 1/2 C grated carrots
1/2 C grated or ground almonds

After grating carrots, put on a board and chop up finely. Make a sauce with 1/2 cup of the carrots and the almonds. Blend together, and pour over the grated carrots. Put in individual bowls with sprouts. Vary this dish by adding other roots -- turnips, beets, parsnips, red or black radish, Jerusalem artichokes. Recipe above for 2.

35

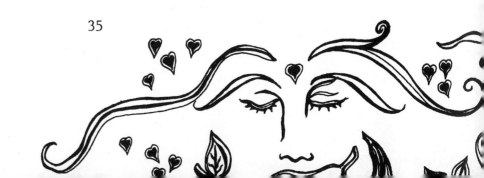

CAULIFLOWER SALAD
WITH CREAMED CASHEW CHEESE

1/2 head cauliflower, cut into bite-size pieces
3 tomatoes, chopped
1/2 red pepper, minced
1/2 C parsley, minced
1 T marjoram

Sauce
1 C ground cashews
1 C rejuvelac
1/2 C grated carrots

Sauce: Allow cashews and rejuvelac to
ferment 4 hours. Then mix with carrots in the
blender.

Salad: Mix vegetables together in attractive serving bowl. Pour sauce over
vegetables before serving. Offer with indoor greens and mixed sprouts.
Serves 4 - 6. Vary this salad by using broccoli instead of cauliflower.

CORN SALAD

1 large ear fresh corn
1 tomato, sliced
1/2 green pepper, chopped
4 T parsley, minced

2 T tamari
1 t coconut oil
1 t kelp
1 t vegetable seasoning

Slice corn off cob, reserve 1/4 cup. Add remaining corn to vegetables
in a bowl, mix. For sauce, add column 2 ingredients to 1/4 cup of corn,
blend together till smooth and creamy. Add rejuvelac if needed. Pour over
salad. For 2.

STUFFED PEPPERS

2 large sweet bell peppers
1 C wheat sprouts
1/4 red pepper, minced
2-3 fresh string beans, chopped
1/4 cup fresh peas from pod
4 T coconut oil
1 T kelp

Hollow out peppers and stuff with mixed ingredients. For 2.

JOSEPH'S SEASONING POWDER

1 1/2 ounce onion powder
1/2 ounce garlic powder
2 ounces comfrey leaf powder, or celery leaf powder, or mixture of both
1 t red cayenne pepper
1 T powdered kelp
1/2 ounce ginger root powder

Mix all these dried ingredients together. Store in tightly capped dark glass jar, and use as a vegetable seasoning.

Make up your own special, individual seasoning powder by combining different types and amounts of spices -- let your taste tell you which ingredients to use!

SEAWEED

Seaweed is very rich in trace elements, minerals (essential to strong bone structure), and iodine (essential to healthy thyroid glands). Seaweed is a wonderful replacement for the salt used so excessively in the typical American diet.

Agar-Agar sticks are made of unbleached seaweed which has been boiled down and dried. These tasteless seaweed bars make a superb substitute for commercial gelatins. Recommended proportions are 4 - 5 cups of liquid to two sticks, stirred together and allowed to sit until thoroughly blended.

SESAME SEEDS

Sesame seed is almost 19 percent protein, compared to the 20 - 30 percent in beef and 13 percent in hard-cooked eggs. It is richly endowed as well with B vitamins and minerals. Whole sesame seeds are also very rich in calcium and iron, while those which have been "decorticated," or husked, have considerably less. Other minerals present in good measure in seeds are potassium, magnesium, and many trace minerals, so you can see that any whole, unprocessed seed will add large amounts of essential food elements to your diet.

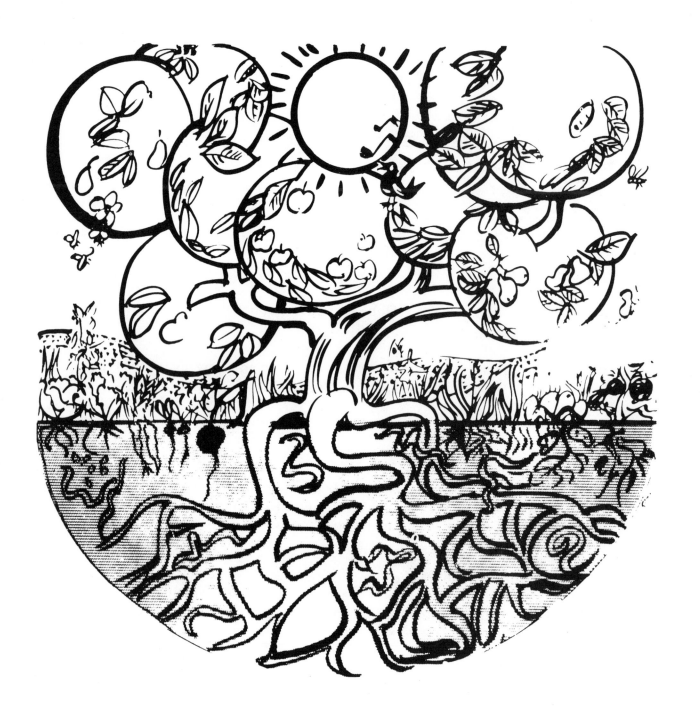

Comment. The experts now tell us that world starvation is only a few years away. This natural tragedy is manmade and is unnecessary if we can as quickly as possible turn back to Nature (God).

Degenerative diseases and all the health problems will at the same time pull back their deadly heads. For over 27 years, work at the Hippocrates Health Institute has proven Nature's ability to clean and heal the body back to normalcy if it is given a chance. Anyone can prove Nature's effectiveness.

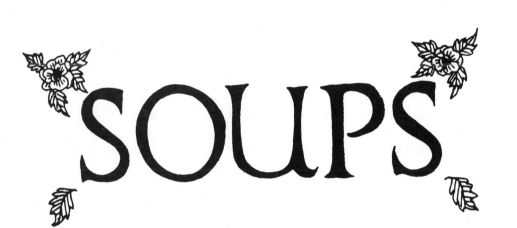

SOUPS

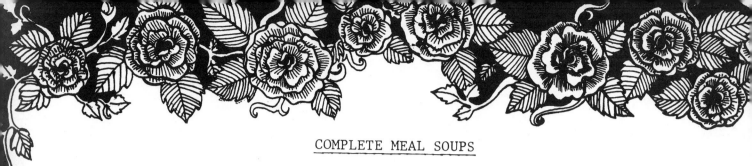

COMPLETE MEAL SOUPS

Complete meal soups are made from sprouts and greens which have been put through the juicer, along with a base (seed yoghurt)* to provide body with needed nourishment. To this mixture can be added various vegetables for flavoring and protein.

The first step is to make a salad of home-grown sprouts, greens, and weeds. The salad can include all kinds of sprouts -- for example, mung bean, lentil, alfalfa, and even a small amount of fenugreek. Even corn and rice can be sprouted. To these sprouts you add a goodly amount of vegetables to the base, for complete nourishment and flavor.

The next step is to flavor the soup. There are all sorts of possibilities. Following are seven favorite complete meal soups:

Number One Soup. This consists of your basic soup, to which unjuiced radish sprouts have been added, along with a base. Two tablespoons of the yoghurt are sufficient for a soupbowl of Number One Soup.

Number Two Soup can be flavored with sauerkraut and mung bean sprouts cut up. The latter should be very juicy and without hulls. A variety of cut-up vegetables can be included, if you wish.

Number Three Soup is basically sprouted sunflower seeds plus one or two tablespoons of yoghurt.

Number Four Soup contains an avocado, which has been crushed into the base. To the soup is added another avocado, cubed or cut into attractive shapes. Some kind of sprouts -- perhaps alfalfa -- makes a good addition.

Number Five Soup should have cut-up tomato and mushrooms, with the addition of sprouts -- any kind that are available and tasty -- or possibly fenugreek sprouts on top of grated carrot.

(NOTE: Always have a little grater on hand at mealtimes to be used at the table by anyone who wants to grate his or her vegetables. Vegetables should be left whole on the table at mealtime because they oxidize very quickly once they are cut up or grated. Therefore, they should be used immediately.)

---

*To prepare the base, use sunflowersesame yoghurt, made from a mixture of sprouted sunflower and sesame seeds (in equal proportions) which have been blended and allowed to ferment at room temperature for about five hours.

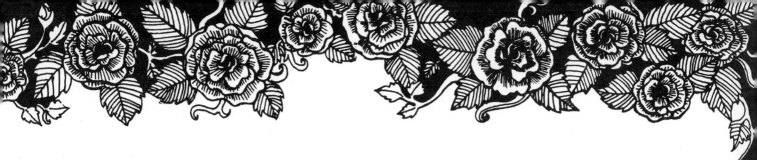

Number Six Soup. This is a useful soup to keep on hand in the refrigerator. It is coconut-flavored, and the coconut used can be grated, cut up, or blended with rejuvelac. (All blended foods should be blended with rejuvelac, to prevent oxidation.)

Number Seven Soup is corn with cucumber which has been peeled and cut up very fine.

All seven soups are extremely easy to digest. Each should contain some sort of sprout or herb for flavoring. You may wish to test-taste these soups while they are being made, to assure a palatable flavor. Serve them with Essene bread to complete the meal.

On days when you have had a soup meal, other meals need not be very large, because a bowl of soup is extremely satisfying. People who are low on energy should have at least two of these soups daily. The complete meal soup is beneficial for all-around well-being, for helping to retain youthfulness, and for helping overcome digestive disorders caused by nutritional deficiencies and unhealthy habits.

Additional suggestions for your complete meal soup are that you add to that nourishment grain crisps, which are very tasty and compatible with the soup. These crisps are made with the dehydrator in various flavors. (See page 20.)

SEED SOUPS

BASIC SEED SOUP

1/2 C seed (sunflower, almond, sesame, pumpkin or sprouted chickpeas)

1-2 C rejuvelac	1 T onion, minced
1 C sprouts	1 T garlic, minced
1 C grated squash: summer, zucchini, hubbard	1/4 t cayenne pepper

Grind seed to a fine powder, and soak in 1 cup of rejuvelac for about 8 hours. Put in blender, and add in sprouts. Blend, adding more rejuvelac for a more liquid texture. Before serving, stir in grated squash and spices. For a more spicy tang, add more onion and garlic, and blend these ingredients into soup instead of stirring in. For a thicker texture, add in more ground seed. For 2 - 4.

Variations: Use different sprouts for different flavors. Try 1/4 cup of radish sprouts for a sharper taste, or 1/2 cup of fenugreek sprouts. Replace the sprouts with indoor greens. Replace the squash with different grated vegetables: beets, parsnips, Jerusalem artichokes, cucumber, or fresh corn off the cob.

GREEN SOUPS

BUCKWHEAT - SPINACH SOUP

1 C chopped buckwheat greens	1/2 avocado
1 C chopped spinach	1-4 cloves garlic
1 medium tomato	2 T kelp

Blend all till creamy: serve over sprouts. For 2.
Variation: For a richer spinach taste, replace buckwheat lettuce with spinach.

GREEN AVOCADO SOUP

1 large, ripe avocado	1 t chives
2 C indoor salad greens	1 t kelp
1 C rejuvelac or spring water	1 t tamari
2 T coconut oil	1/4 C sunflower seed meal

Blend greens, fluid and seasonings. For extra thickening add the ground seed, or an additional avocado. Buckwheat is an excellent choice for indoor greens. Serves 2-4.

WINTER SOUP MEAL

1 C indoor greens

1 C chopped watercress

1/2 C sunflower seed meal

1/2 C water or rejuvelac

2-4 T onion, minced

1/4 t cayenne pepper

Blend ingredients to a smooth consistency. Pour over sunflower greens, mung sprouts and dulse. For 2 - 4.

Variation: Use a comfrey - buckwheat lettuce - mustard green combination. Leave out the cayenne if you do use mustard greens.

VEGETABLE SOUPS

VEGETABLE SOUP

1 tomato

1/2 small cucumber

1/4 beet, sliced

1 small green onion, sliced

1/4 small potato, sliced

2-3 cabbage leaves

2-3 spinach or chard leaves

1/2 C rejuvelac or water

1 t vegetable seasoning

1/4 t dulse

Blend all until smooth and creamy. Any vegetables in season may be used. For 4 - 6.

COMFREY - CARROT SOUP

15 medium sized comfrey leaves

1 C carrot juice

1/2 avocado

1 small zucchini, chopped

Blend ingredients and serve over greens and sprouts. For 2.

Variations: Try celery or cabbage juice or any other green juice in place of the carrot. Add in a few T of sauerkraut.

43

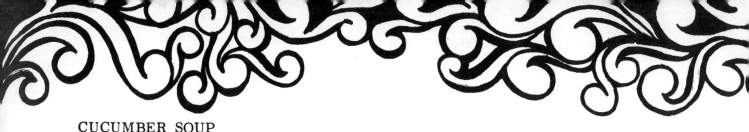

CUCUMBER SOUP

1 C cucumber, grated
2 C seed milk
2 T green onions, slivered

1 T kelp
8-12 cucumber slices
4 T fresh chives

Combine grated cucumber, seed milk. Serve in individual bowls decorated with cucumber slices, onions and chives. Sprinkle the kelp on top. For 2.

ASPARAGUS SOUP

2 C raw asparagus, chopped
2 C indoor salad greens
1/2 C almond meal

2 stalks celery, chopped
2 sprigs parsley, minced
1 T coconut oil

Save asparagus tips to top soup with. Blend all other ingredients. Add in almond meal bit by bit. Serve over a bed of alfalfa sprouts. For 4.

CAULIFLOWER SOUP

1/2 head cauliflower, chopped
1 avocado
1 C celery, chopped
1/2-1 C rejuvelac

1/4 C radish sprouts
1 T kelp
1/2 lemon, juiced
1 t savory

Blend all ingredients to desired consistency. Serve over alfalfa or mung sprouts. For 4.

CREAM OF PEA SOUP

1 C fresh garden peas
1 C almond or cashew milk
1/2 C carrot juice

1/2 C diced avocado
1 t herbal seasoning
1 t tamari

Add all ingredients to blender; blend till creamy.
Gently stir in a few extra peas after blending.
For 2. Vary this recipe by using a cup of
        grated squash,
          or chopped
            okra.

44

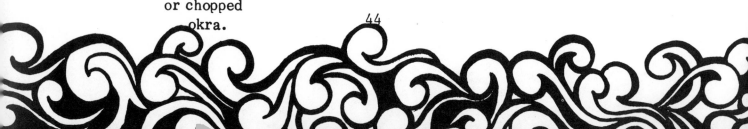

RAW CELERY SOUP #1

1/2 C fresh celery juice
1/2 C fresh carrot juice
1/2 lemon, squeezed

1/2 tomato, chopped
2-4 T minced pepper
2-4 T minced onion
2-4 T minced celery
1 clove garlic, pressed

1 t each: almond meal, sesame meal, coconut oil

Blend juices and meal till creamy, then add in oil. Add in finely chopped vegetables for taste and texture. For 2.

RAW CELERY SOUP #2

1 small bunch celery
1 small zucchini
2 small potatoes
1 small onion

2 C celery-carrot juice
2 T minced parsley
1 T coconut oil
1 T tamari

Dice the vegetables well; add all to blender bit by bit, reserving the juice and a few celery greens for topping. When you have a smooth, soupy texture, (adding in a bit more oil for thickness if need be), fold in celery-carrot juice. Toss celery greens over each bowl. For 6 - 8.

Variation: Add shredded beets as a colorful topping.
Leave some vegetables unblended, so the soup has a more crunchy texture.
Make this a squash soup by substituting 2 summer squashes for the bunch of celery.
Give this soup a healthy tang by using 2 cups of fresh sauerkraut juice.

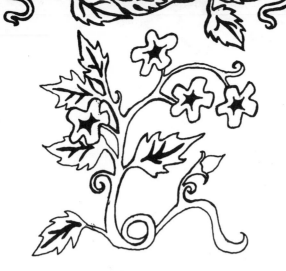

CORN
SOUPS

UNCOOKED CORN CHOWDER

2 medium tomatoes, chopped
1/2 C rejuvelac or water
1 large ear fresh corn
1/2 C sunflower seed sprouts
2 C alfalfa sprouts

Blend tomatoes and water, and add in the corn, cut off the cob. Pour over individual bowls of alfalfa sprouts. Top with sunflower sprouts. For 2.

CORN CHOWDER WITH VEGETABLES

2 ears fresh corn	4 green onions, chopped	1 T sunflower meal
2 medium tomatoes	1 diced avocado	1 T coconut oil
1 C shredded zucchini	1/2 bell pepper, chopped	1 T kelp
	1 C carrot juice	

Cut the corn from the cob and place in blender, but save a few kernels to sprinkle on top of each bowl. Scrape the cob with the back of the knife for extra juice. Add all the ingredients and blend. Serves 4 - 6.

CORN SOUP WITH MUSHROOMS

1 C fresh corn, cut from cob   1/2 C sliced mushrooms
1 C spring water or rejuvelac   1/4 C chopped kale
1/2 C bean sprouts   1 T kelp

Blend the corn and water. Add the remaining ingredients.
Serve over indoor greens.

Variations: Use different kinds of bean sprouts.
    Try curly endive instead of kale, or any
    other green.
    Make a soup
    with just
    corn and
    one
    green.

46

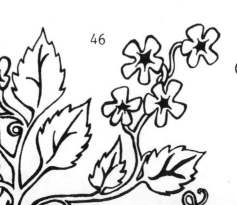

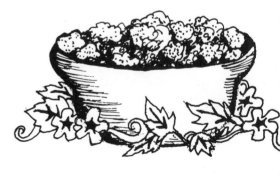

BEET SOUPS

BEET REJUVELAC SOUP

1 large beet, diced	1/2 avocado
1 C rejuvelac	1 lemon, juiced
1 clove garlic, pressed	2 T pink sauerkraut

Blend garlic and beet with rejuvelac. Reduce to a creamy consistency. Add in other ingredients, and blend. Before serving, add 2 T sauerkraut. Serve over chopped sunflower greens. Serves 2 - 4.

BORSCHT #1

2 C shredded beets	1 small green onion, chopped
1-2 C rejuvelac	1-2 T tamari
1/2 C almond meal	1 t thyme

Blend all to a smooth consistency. Serve over indoor greens and sprouts. 2 - 4.

BORSCHT #2

4 small or 2 large beets	1 medium potato
1/4 head medium cabbage	1 stick celery
1 - 1 1/2 C rejuvelac	1 scallion

Scrub and dice the beets. Shred the cabbage, chop other vegetables. Blend all vegetables a bit at a time, so your blender doesn't become overloaded. Save a few T's of shredded beet to sprinkle on each bowl. Serves 4 - 6.

Variations: Substitute any other root vegetable(s) -- turnip, parsnip, Jerusalem artichoke -- in any of these beet soup recipes.
In place of rejuvelac, try a cup of juiced greens, or carrot juice.

SPROUT SOUPS

LENTIL-ONION SOUP

2 C sprouted lentils	1/2 C buckwheat lettuce, chopped
1 C rejuvelac	1/2 C minced onion
1/2 C parsley, minced	2 T coconut oil
1/2 C celery, minced	1 t sweet basil

Blend all! Use this as a full meal. For 4 – 6.

Variations: Blend in a medium-sized sliced potato, for a thicker
            soup. Add in a clove of pressed garlic for more zest.
            Top the soup with more lentil sprouts and minced onion.

LENTIL SOUP

2 C lentil sprouts	1 celery stalk
2 medium tomatoes	1 small zucchini
1 small onion	2 T parsley, minced
1 small pepper	2 T vegetable seasoning

Chop or mince vegetables. Blend tomatoes first, add in other vegetables, saving
some to add in for crunchiness. Put lentils in blender last, so they are barely
chopped. Serve over chopped indoor greens. For 4 – 6.

CHICK PEA SPROUT SOUP

1 C sprouted chick peas	1 C grated squash: summer, zucchini
1-2 C rejuvelac	2-4 T minced onion
2 C alfalfa-fenugreek sprouts	1-2 T kelp

Chop chick pea sprouts a bit, then blend with rejuvelac and all other ingredients.
Serve over sprouts or indoor greens. For 2 – 4.

TOMATO SOUPS

SUMMER TREAT

3 large tomatoes
2 large cucumbers
1 sweet red pepper, finely chopped
1 T minced onion
1 T minced parsley or watercress
1 T kelp
1 T dill

At a slow speed, blend the tomatoes, and 1 - 1/2 cucumbers. Add in the pepper, onion, kelp, dill. Before serving, float in the remaining cucumber, finely sliced. Garnish with parsley. For 4 - 6.

TOMATO SOUP

3-4 medium tomatoes
2-3 T green chives, minced
1 t each: sweet basil, thyme
1 t coconut oil

1/2 C carrot juice
1/2 C celery juice
1/2 C beet or potato juice
juice of 1/2 lemon

Liquefy tomatoes in blender. Add in chives, spices and oil. Stir in juices by hand, and serve over indoor greens. For 4.

TOMATO CREAM SOUP

2 ripe tomatoes
1 C rejuvelac
15 comfrey leaves
1/2 cucumber, sliced
1 stalk celery

1 green pepper
4 sprigs parsley
1 clove garlic
1 T kelp
1 avocado

Blend all ingredients (except avocado) with the rejuvelac to a smooth consistency. Add the avocado, and reblend. This will make a complete meal for 4 - 6. Use any wild edible in place of the comfrey.

TOMATO-SQUASH SOUP

4 medium tomatoes
2 C grated zucchini
2 C grated yellow squash
1 chopped leek or onion
1 C almond meal
2 T kelp

Blend all, except for approximately 1 cup of combined vegetables. Float these in, and serve over sprouts. For 4 - 6.

TOMATO-AVOCADO CHOWDER

3 medium tomatoes	1 whole avocado, diced
1/2 C grated carrots	1 small onion, chopped
1/2 C grated celery	1 small bell pepper, chopped
1/2 C grated cabbage	1 T kelp

Blend tomatoes and avocado. Add in remaining ingredients and blend very briefly to keep the thick, chowdery consistency. For 4 - 6.

Variation: Use carrot and celery juice (1/2 cup each), and replace the cabbage with sauerkraut.

POTATO SOUPS

POTATO-MUSHROOM SOUP

2 medium potatoes, unpeeled, grated	1 T each: paprika
2 C cashew milk (2/3 C cashews,	tamari
2 C water, blended)	1 C chopped onions
3 C chopped mushrooms	2 medium tomatoes, chopped

Blend all ingredients, saving onions and tomatoes to float into the soup. For 4 - 6.

To thicken any vegetable soup, blend in avocado, ground seed meal, or coconut oil.

POTATO-TOMATO SOUP

1 medium potato, grated.   1 stalk celery, chopped
1 medium tomato, chopped   1/4 C radish sprouts

Blend all. For 1. Served over individual bowls of sprouts -- for 2.

POTATO-BROCCOLI SOUP

2 medium potatoes, grated   1/4 head broccoli
1/2 C rejuvelac   3-4 T coconut oil

Cut off broccoli flowerettes, and chop tender portions of broccoli stalks. Blend the stalks with the grated potato and rejuvelac, until all is creamy. Then float in broccoli flowerettes and serve. For 2.

POTATO-ENDIVE SOUP

1 medium potato, grated   1/4 C rejuvelac
8-12 leaves endive, chopped   1/4 t cayenne pepper

Blend the potato and rejuvelac, add in endive and pepper. For 2.
For variety, use different weeds and greens, and leave some pieces whole.

POTATO-SAUERKRAUT SOUP

1 medium potato, grated   1/4 C rejuvelac
2 C sauerkraut (see page 8)   1 clove garlic, pressed

Blend all. For 2. Make this thicker by adding in 1 cup of fermented seed sauce.

POTATO-CELERY SOUP

1 medium potato   1/4 C rejuvelac
2 C celery, chopped   1 avocado

Blend potato with rejuvelac and 1-1/2 cups of celery. Add in avocado, and blend.
Pour over sprouts in individual bowls, and top with remaining celery. For 2 - 4.

Variations: In place of the potato in any of these soups, try beet, turnip, parsnip
              or any root vegetable.
              Add in radishes, mustard greens, garlic for additional flavors.

FRUIT SOUPS

Soup for a meal? These easily prepared soups, with their combination of flavors make delightful, refreshing meals, especially on summer days. They are all natural sweets. Use regional fruits in season, referring to the food combining chart in the back of this book. For a chunky texture, blend some fruits, and leave some in bits. Decorate these tasty soups with currants, grapes, banana slices, or whole slices of the fruits you've blended fanned out in a circular design. Increase, decrease the amounts called for as you desire. With fruit, it all tastes delicious!

COMPANY FRUIT SOUP

1 quart fresh ripe fruit, pitted and diced
    (try any combination of sweet and sub-acid: cherries, peaches, apricots, grapes, mangoes, plums, nectarines, bananas, etc.)
2 cups berries
    (pick one or any combination of strawberries, blueberries, raspberries, boysenberries, blackberries, etc.)

1 apple, cored and diced	1 pear, cored and diced
2 t cinnamon	2 t ginger

Blend, and decorate with grapes and berries, or sliced bananas. For 6 - 8. When blending, fill blender to halfway mark, to avoid overloading. Make this in batches, and stir all together before serving.

AMBROSIA FRUIT SOUP

1 cup concord grapes	1 cup coconut
1 cup green grapes	1/2 t cinnamon
1 cup chopped tart apples (Pippin)	1 nectarine, sectioned

Remove grape seeds; blend grapes to sauce consistency. Blend in apples and add cinnamon to taste. Pour into individual serving bowls, and decorate with nectarine slices. For 4.

LIQUIFIED FRUIT SOUP

1 cup fresh apple juice	1/2 cup coconut milk
1 cup fresh fruit pieces (sub-acid)	1/2 cup whole berries

Blend well and pour into soup cups. Serve with a few berries floating on top. 2 - 4. Use rejuvelac if coconut milk is unavailable.

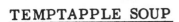

TEMPTAPPLE SOUP

4 ripe apples (any variety)
1/2-1 C apple cider or rejuvelac
1/2-1 t cinnamon

Blend apples and cinnamon, adding liquid as needed. For 2.
Variation: Add in nectarines, fresh apricots or figs, plums.

FRESH FIG SOUP

3-4 fresh figs, chopped   1/2-1 C rejuvelac
1-2 peaches, chopped   1 t ginger or cinnamon
1/2 C fried apricots, soaked and diced   1/4 C grated coconut

Blend these fruits together, saving some peach slices for decoration. If you find
fresh apricots, use them in the same proportion as the figs, and substitute prunes in
place of the apricots. For 2.

COCONUT-DATE SOUP

1 coconut   1 C blueberries (optional)
1 C rejuvelac   1 C grapes (optional)
1 C dates, soaked

Open coconut (use coconut water for another fruit soup). Break meat into inch cubes.
Put rejuvelac in blender, and slowly add the coconut cubes. Finally add in soaked
dates and blend to a sauce consistency. If the blender is filled over two-thirds, start
a new batch. This is a very rich soup. Float in berries and grapes if desired, or
serve them in a separate bowl, and let your diners add them in. For 4 - 6.

Variation: Offer your diners a choice of fruits to add into their soup. A variety of
            sub-acid fruits provides good combinations since the coconut-date base is so
            sweet. Try apples, peaches, pears, nectarines, cherries or fresh apricots.

MELON SOUP

1/2 cantalope
1/2 honeydew melon
2 C watermelon chunks, deseeded
2 C watermelon juice

Blend all lightly. For 4.

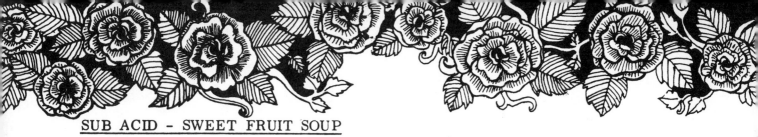

SUB ACID - SWEET FRUIT SOUP

1 C chopped fresh peaches
1 C chopped apples (leave skins on)
1 C chopped fresh pears

1/2 C dried apricots, soaked
2 bananas
1/4 t cinnamon or ginger

Soak apricots at least 4 hours. Save soak water to thin soup with, if needed. Blend ingredients, reserving 6-8 banana slices for decoration of bowls. Raisins are another tasty decoration. For 2 - 4.

RAPPLE SOUP

4 large delicious apples, cored
1/2 C rejuvelac (approximately)

1 1/2 C raisins, soaked
1/4 t cinnamon

Chop up 3 of the apples, and grate 1. Blend the chopped apples with raisins and a bit of the rejuvelac. Add in cinnamon and enough rejuvelac to get a smooth consistency. Before serving in individual bowls, stir in the grated apple. For 2 - 4.

Variations: Add in 1/4 cup grated coconut. Use dates or figs in place of raisins, or any dried fruit, for example, prunes.

BERRY DELICIOUS SOUP

2 C ripe berries: strawberries, blueberries, raspberries, blackberries, boysenberries, huckleberries
1/2 C coconut milk, or rejuvelac
1 t freshly ground ginger root

Blend berries till smooth, saving some to float on top. Add liquid to thin, if needed. Enjoy! For 2.

CHEERY CHERRY SOUP

2 C fresh cherries, pitted
1 large peach, sliced
1/2-1 C cold spring water, or rejuvelac

Blend these fresh fruits to a smooth consistency, adding liquid if necessary. Let a few cherry pieces decorate this colorful soup. For 2 - 4.
        For variation, add in a fresh plum.

TREATS
OF LIFE

DATES, FIGS, AND HONEY

Dates: Dates are among those fruits which are richest in natural carbohydrates. Date sugar is a very good substitute for cane or other sugars, and dates are therefore one of the most valuable replacements for candy. Because their carbohydrate content is composed of natural sugars, dates are compatible with other fruits. They make a useful replacement for bread and other starches.

Figs: Fresh figs, both white and dark, are exceedingly beneficial, being, in fact, one of the best natural laxatives. They contain nearly 80 percent water and have a very high potassium, calcium, and magnesium content.

Honey: Honey is a delicious and popular as well as valuable food, containing natural vitamins and minerals -- such as B_6, thiamine, riboflavin, and vitamin C -- as well as a most important component: dextrose (a sugar of the glucose group). Dextrose is quickly absorbed by the upper intestinal tract and goes directly to the brain and muscles, where is it converted into glycogen and used in the body to dispel fatigue. Not only is honey one of Nature's energy boosters, it also is known to be good for skin blemishes and a good preservative for some foods. Some researchers also say that honey is valuable for prolonging life.

Unheated, unfiltered honey is the only kind of natural sugar which can safely be stored in the liver and muscles. If you see that crystals are forming in the honey you buy, you can be sure that it's good. Always look for labels that say, "Uncooked (or unheated), unfiltered natural honey."

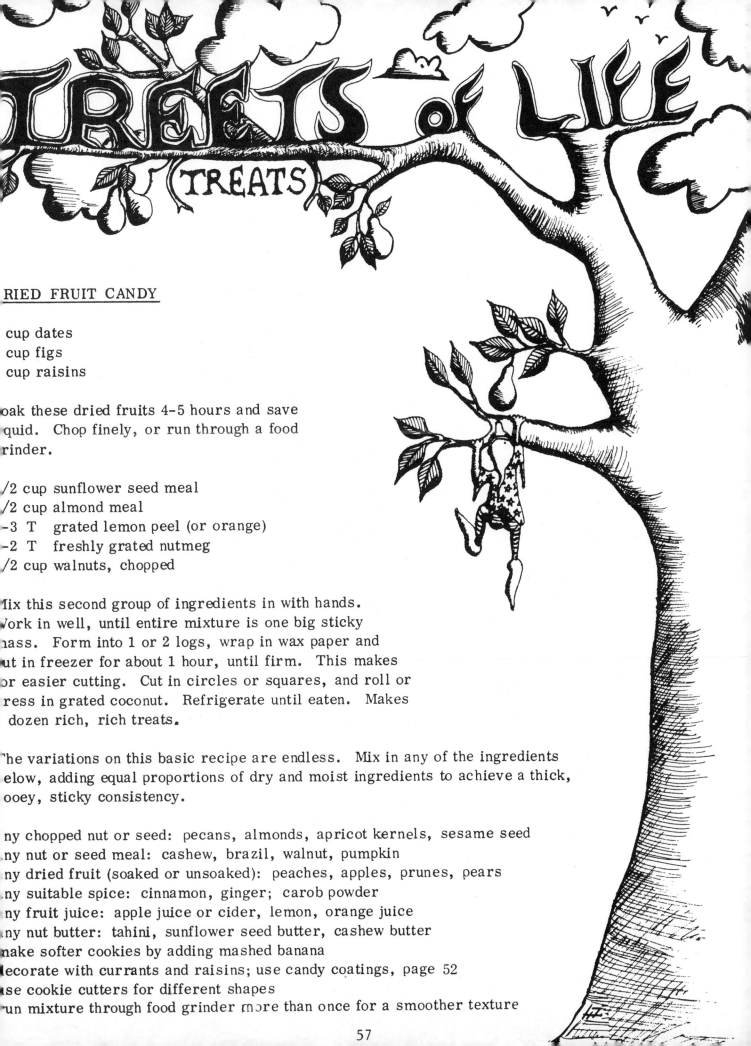

TREES OF LIFE
(TREATS)

RIED FRUIT CANDY

cup dates
cup figs
cup raisins

oak these dried fruits 4-5 hours and save
quid. Chop finely, or run through a food
rinder.

/2 cup sunflower seed meal
/2 cup almond meal
-3 T   grated lemon peel (or orange)
-2 T   freshly grated nutmeg
/2 cup walnuts, chopped

Mix this second group of ingredients in with hands.
Work in well, until entire mixture is one big sticky
mass. Form into 1 or 2 logs, wrap in wax paper and
ut in freezer for about 1 hour, until firm. This makes
or easier cutting. Cut in circles or squares, and roll or
ress in grated coconut. Refrigerate until eaten. Makes
 dozen rich, rich treats.

he variations on this basic recipe are endless. Mix in any of the ingredients
elow, adding equal proportions of dry and moist ingredients to achieve a thick,
ooey, sticky consistency.

ny chopped nut or seed: pecans, almonds, apricot kernels, sesame seed
ny nut or seed meal: cashew, brazil, walnut, pumpkin
ny dried fruit (soaked or unsoaked): peaches, apples, prunes, pears
ny suitable spice: cinnamon, ginger; carob powder
ny fruit juice: apple juice or cider, lemon, orange juice
ny nut butter: tahini, sunflower seed butter, cashew butter
nake softer cookies by adding mashed banana
ecorate with currants and raisins; use candy coatings, page 52
se cookie cutters for different shapes
un mixture through food grinder more than once for a smoother texture

CAROB RAISIN GOODIES

1 C carob powder   2 t uncooked vanilla extract
1 C coconut oil   1/2 C spring water
1/2 C raw honey   1 1/2 C raisins, chopped

Mix carob, oil, honey, vanilla and water. Add in chopped raisins and mix again. Form into small patties. Makes about 2 dozen.

CASHEW BUTTER BALLS

8 T raw cashew butter (1/2 C)   1 C cashew pieces
1 C each: raisins, pitted dates   3/4 C grated coconut

Put dates and raisins through a food grinder on a medium setting, or soak and mince finely. Mix well with 3/4 cup coconut and cashew butter. Add in cashew pieces. Form into balls and roll in additional coconut.

DATE-PECAN SQUARES

2 C pitted dates   1 1/2 C dried coconut
1/2 C pecans   1 t uncooked vanilla extract

Run dates and pecans through a food chopper, or mince by hand. Sprinkle 1/2 of the coconut on a plate. Place the date-pecan mixture on this and tamp down well, so that coconut is absorbed into the date mat. Sprinkle the remaining coconut on top and tamp again. Cut into squares and wrap in waxed paper, or store in a jar. Refrigerate until needed. Makes 8-12 squares.

Variation: Try a dried fig-cashew combination. Raisin-almond is also good. Either of these variations can be used as a pie crust for a raw fruit pie.

RAISIN-WALNUT PATTIES

1 C each: raisins, walnuts, cashew meal, dried coconut
2-3 T fresh (unsprayed) orange peel

Grind ingredients, mix well, and form into patties.

58

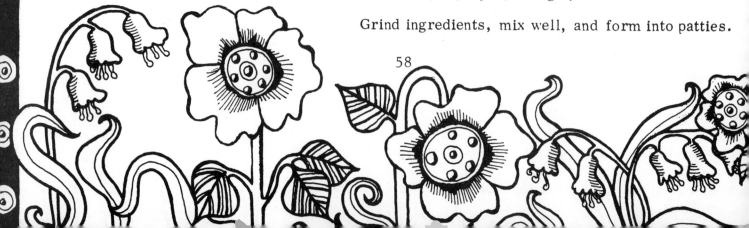

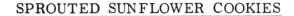

SPROUTED SUNFLOWER COOKIES

2 C sprouted sunflower seeds
1 C soft dates, pitted
1 C raisins, soaked

2 T nut butter
2 T organic orange peel
1 T vanilla extract (pure)

Place seeds, dates, raisins on a wooden board and chop well. Add nut butter, peelings, and extract. Form into balls and/or other creative shapes. Will make about 1 1/2 dozen small cookies.

Variations: Put sprouted seeds, dates and raisins through a food grinder for a more smooth consistency.

Use almonds, pecans, brazil nuts and figs instead of sunflower seeds and dates. Grind some nuts into a meal, and chop the rest.

Add in more nut butter, and decrease amount of dates or raisins.

Top the cookies with sesame seeds.

Use cinnamon or carob powder in place of, or in addition to the vanilla.

Instead of forming into balls, mold whole dough into one large block and refrigerate. Use as a raw pie crust, or cut into pick-up energy bars.

CAROB FUDGE BALLS

1 C sesame butter
1 C raisins
1/2 C unsweetened coconut, grated

4 T raw carob powder
1 T raw honey
1/4 t vanilla

Stir all ingredients together. Form into balls. Makes about 1 1/2 dozen small balls. Refrigerate.

PEANUT BUTTER BALLS

1/2 C raw peanut butter
1/2 C raw honey

1/2 C sunflower seed meal
1/2 C raisins, chopped

Mix all together; form into little balls. Makes about 2 dozen little goodies.

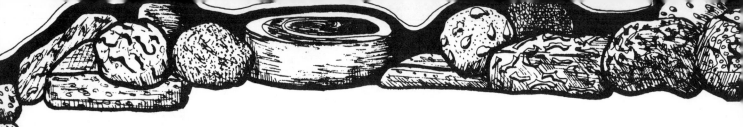

SUNFLOWER SESAME TREATS

3/4 C sunflower seed meal
1/4 C tahini
1/2 C unsweetened shredded coconut

1/4 C raw honey
1/3 C raw wheat germ
1 C dates or raisins, chopped

Combine ingredients in order given. Mix all together thoroughly. Separate mixture into two portions; roll into logs. Wrap each in wax paper and store in refrigerator. When chilled, remove and cut into 1/2 inch pieces. Serve as a snack or with fresh fruit as a dessert. Yield: two 4-inch rolls.

FIG BARS

2 C black figs, soaked and minced
1 C coconut, freshly grated or dried

1 T raw honey
1 t pure vanilla extract

Combine all ingredients well, form into bars or any other shape. Refrigerate until enjoyed. Yield: approximately 1 dozen bars.

Variation: Add 1 cup of nut meal, or coarsely chopped nuts in place of the coconut, and use coconut to dust the bars.
Add freshly ground nutmeg, lemon peel.

SUNFLOWER SEED CANDY

2 C sunflower seeds
2 T pure vanilla extract
1 T each: honey, coconut oil, nut butter
extra coconut oil, as needed

Makes about 1 dozen balls.

Variation: Roll in coating mixtures outlined on next page.
Try different seed meals: cashew, pumpkin, pecan, brazil, pignolia.

Blend sunflower seeds to a fine powder. Blend with the cover on, then remove cover and push seeds down and under blades with a spatula. Divide the meal into 2 bowls.

To one, add 1 T honey, oil, and vanilla. To the other, add 1 heaping T nut butter and vanilla. Form into balls, adding oil if needed for texture.

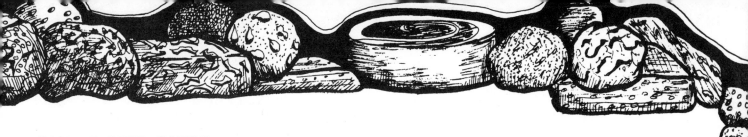

SESAME SEED CANDY

2 C sesame seeds
1/2 C coconut oil
2 T honey

1/2 t vanilla
1 T peanut butter (heaping T)
1 T carob

Start the blender with oil. Gradually, add in sesame seeds. Help push seeds down and under the blades. Add honey and vanilla to the mixture and continue blending until smooth. Divide mixture into three bowls: add peanut butter to one, carob to the next, and leave one plain. Shape into balls. Makes 1 - 1 1/2 dozen candies.

SESAME SEED TAFFY

2 C sesame seeds
1 C coconut oil

2 T each: honey, vanilla
1 t each: almond extract, carob

Put oil in blender and gradually add in sesame seeds. Let it run until mixture gets hot and looks glossy. Add in flavorings. Turn mixture out into a bowl, and with a rubber spatula, knead it up on the side of the bowl, squeezing out the oil. Finish this kneading with your hands. Roll dough into a log, slice. Decorate with seed candy coatings outlined on the next page. Makes about 1 dozen patties.

PUMPKIN SEED CANDY

2 C pumpkin seeds
1/2 C oil (from sesame
      seed taffy above)
2 T honey
1/2 t pure vanilla
1/2 t almond extract
1/2 t lemon juice
      (optional)

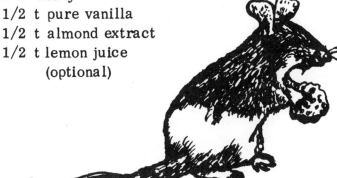

Chop nuts well -- by hand, in nut and seed grinder, or in blender. They needn't all be the same consistency. Mix all ingredients well, and form into patties or roll into balls. Coat with mixtures listed on following page. For storage, place between sheets of waxed paper in freezer, or in refrigerator. Makes about 1- 1 1/2 dozen balls.

Variations: All these candies are variations on the same theme. Create your own special treat. You need only keep the same proportion of nuts to oil (4 to 1).

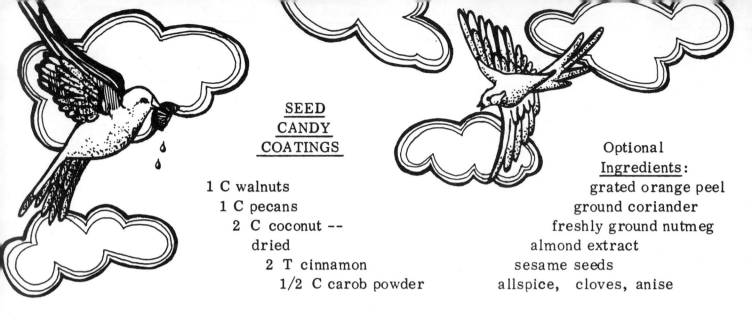

SEED
CANDY
COATINGS

1 C walnuts
1 C pecans
2 C coconut --
dried
2 T cinnamon
1/2 C carob powder

Optional
Ingredients:
grated orange peel
ground coriander
freshly ground nutmeg
almond extract
sesame seeds
allspice, cloves, anise

Chop nuts in blender, turning blender on and off quickly until you have a very fine, powdery consistency. You could also use a nut and seed grinder, or a grain mill.

Separate the nuts into 2 bowls; leave one plain, add the cinnamon to the other. Divide the coconut into 2 bowls; add 2 T carob to one; leave the other plain. Put the remaining carob powder in another bowl.

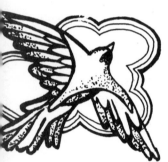

These are your seed candy coatings -- dip the dried fruit or nut candies into a bowl, making sure the coating adheres by pressing and tamping the candies into the coatings.

Save these coatings in tightly covered glass jars or plastic bags. The amounts given will coat about 3 dozen small candies.

Variations: Use different nuts. Add in optional ingredients. Grind nuts more or less coarsely. Combine cinnamon and carob. Combine coconut and cinnamon.

COCONUT KISS

1 medium coconut
1-2 C seed meal (cashew, almond, sunflower)

4-6 T unfiltered honey
1 C pecan meats

Remove shell and peel from the fresh coconut, reserving liquid (use in a fruit soup). Grate coconut meat and blend with honey. Turn into a bowl. Add in seed meal until you have a thick consistency that will form balls. Roll balls in extra seed meal, or use candy coatings above. Place a pecan meat on the top of each kiss. Makes about 2 dozen.

To grate coconut: - Chop up with a knife, and chop more finely in blender
- Put pieces through Champion juicer, using homogenizing blank
- Grate by hand
- Put pieces through a food grinder or salad maker

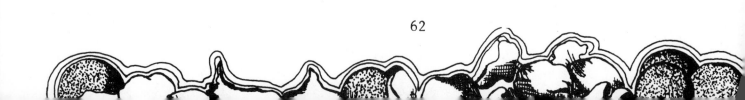

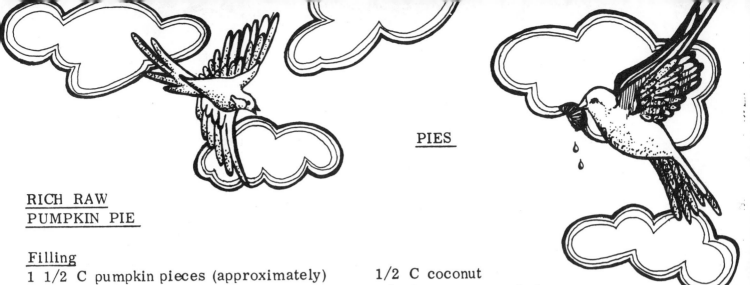

PIES

RICH RAW
PUMPKIN PIE

Filling
1 1/2 C pumpkin pieces (approximately)
1 C cashew pieces
2-4 T fresh orange or lemon juice
2 T unfiltered honey

1/2 C coconut
1/4 C raisins, soaked

Blend column 1 ingredients, then add coconut and raisins. If filling is too thick, blend in more pumpkin pieces and fruit juice. If filling is too thin, add more ground nuts. The mixture will firm up when refrigerated, but it should have a thick, pancake batter kind of texture before being chilled.

Crust
1 1/2 - 2 C cashew pieces
2 C rejuvelac or spring water
1/2 C grated coconut

3-4 T raw honey
3-4 T cashew nut butter
1-2 C sunflower seed
         meal

Blend cashews and rejuvelac (or water). Add into blender grated coconut, honey and nut butter. Turn into a bowl, and mix in seed meal bit by bit to gain a thick, doughy texture. Then press into a pie plate, and add filling. Makes enough for 1 large pie. If this is too much for your pie tin, turn to one of your old frying pans. Refrigerate 4 hours to set.

KANTI'S RAW FRUIT PIE

Filling
10-12 tart green apples, cored
1 C raisins or currants

1 T cinnamon
juice of 1 medium lemon

Grate 1/2 of the apples, blend the other half. Mix in the remaining ingredients.

Crust
1 pound soft dates, pitted
1/2 pound walnuts, ground to a flour

3/4 C coconut, shredded

Knead all together. Press into a 10" pie plate and pour in filling. Decorate.

63

RAW FRUIT PIE

1 C raisins	1 C nuts, coarsely ground
1 C dates, pitted	1/2 C unfiltered honey
1/2 C grated orange peel	1 t cinnamon

Grind up the raisins, dates and orange skins. Mix in all the other ingredients, and place in a pie plate. Refrigerate before serving. This does not need a crust. Makes 1 small pie.

Decorations

1 banana, sliced	1/4 C grated coconut
1 handful grapes	1 apple, cored and sliced
1 pear, sliced	1/4 C raisins
1 peach, sliced	1 nectarine, sliced
whole or coarsely chopped nuts	sliced almonds
flowers	grated orange or lemon peel
cherries, whole berries	mint leaves

Use fresh fruit to make a pleasing design on top of your pies. Make circles and scalloped circular patterns with the edges of the sliced fruits. Use raisins for the centers of the patterns, if you like. Grated coconut sprinkled over a pie gives a pleasing effect.

DATE PIE

Filling

4 grated apples	1/2 C shredded coconut
2 mashed bananas	1/2 C almond meal

Mix grated apples, bananas, dates. Add coconut and almond meal slowly, cutting back on almond meal if necessary. Mix to a pudding consistency, so filling does not run when cut.

Crust

2 C dates	3/4 C coconut	1/4 C carob powder

Soak dates in spring water approximately 12 hours. Save water for a fruit soup, or add to filling above. Pit dates and put through a food grinder, or use mortar and pestle to make a paste. Add coconut and carob powder to make a spreadable mixture. Press into a pie plate. Spoon filling into crust. Refrigerate 2 hours to allow pie to set. Garnish with apple slices just before serving.

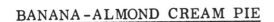

BANANA-ALMOND CREAM PIE

Filling

3 bananas

1/2 - 1 C rejuvelac or spring water

2 C almond meal

1 t cinnamon or nutmeg

Blend almonds and bananas in roughly equal parts. Add enough rejuvelac to attain a thick, pudding consistency. Freeze until firm (1-2 hours).

Crust

1 C almonds, finely ground

1 C raisins, soaked 1 hour

1 C black figs, soaked 1 hour

1/2 t ground cloves

Mix all together. Press into a pie plate. Add the frozen filling; decorate and serve.

BANANA CREAM PIE

4-5 bananas

1/2 C apple juice

1 C grated coconut

2 t tahini

2 t honey

1 t pure vanilla extract

Mash 2 of the bananas, put in blender with the apple juice, 1/2 cup of coconut, and the other ingredients. Blend till smooth. Slice the remaining 2 or 3 bananas, and gently mix in with the last 1/2 cup of coconut. This will make a 10" pie.

For a crust, see page 58. Date-Pecan Squares, or the Raisin-Walnut Patties. The crust given in the preceding pie recipe will also work well.

When decorating this pie, include raisins or currants, apple slices and coconut.

MINCE PIE

1 C raisins, soaked

1 C dates: soaked, pitted, chopped

1 C grated apple

1 T raw honey

1 t cinnamon

1/2 t each: nutmeg, cloves

Mix ingredients together. This pie really doesn't need a crust. Yield: 1 8-inch pie.

Variations: To lighten this rich pie, add in more grated (or chopped) fruit: plums, nectarines, peaches, fresh pineapple. Try blending some of the fruit before mixing in, for a thinner texture.

RAW CARROT CAKE

I
1/2 C soy flour
1/2 C sunflower seed meal
1/2 C raw wheat germ
1/2 C bran
1/2 C steel cut rolled oats
1/2 C shredded coconut
2 t kelp
1 t cinnamon
1 t nutmeg

II 8 T almond butter (use heaping T's)
4 T raw honey
3 T coconut oil
3 T water
1 t vanilla extract

III 1/2 C raisins, soaked
1/2 C soft dates, soaked
1/2 C shredded coconut
3 C shredded or ground carrots

66

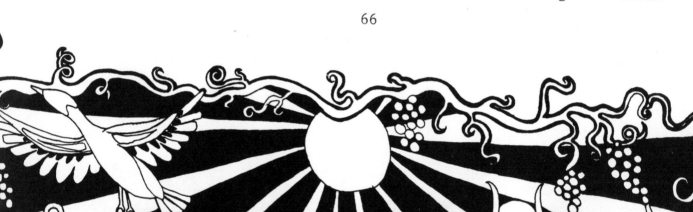

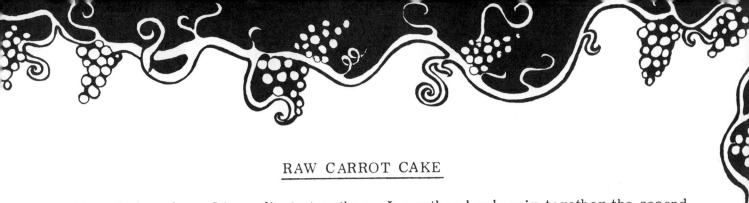

RAW CARROT CAKE

Mix all the column I ingredients together. In another bowl, mix together the second group of ingredients. Grind through food grinder the soaked raisins and dates and carrots (or chop extremely finely and blend; or homogenize with Champion juicer).

Mix fried fruit and carrots with the honey mixture; then mix with dry ingredients. Put through the food grinder a second time. This is important -- it gives the loaf a lighter texture. If you are not using a food grinder, mix all ingredients very well with a spoon, adding spring water if needed.

Form into a loaf pan that has been well oiled.* Refrigerate for several hours before unmolding. Garnish with coconut. Makes 1 large loaf cake.

* with coconut oil.   67

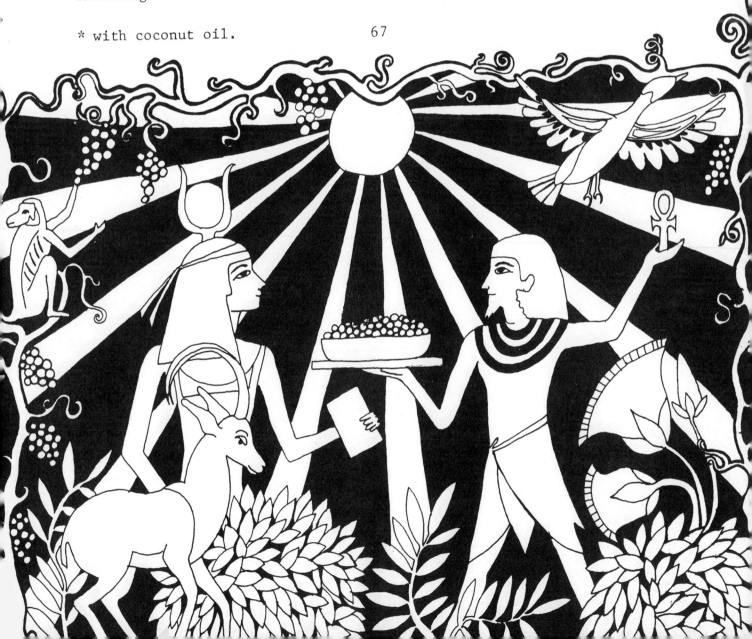

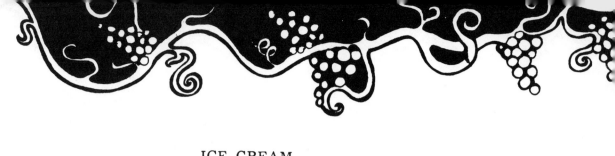

ICE CREAM

BANANA ICE CREAM #1

8-10 bananas

Peel bananas and freeze 24 hours, until quite solid. Just before serving, run them through the Champion juicer, with the homogenizing plate in. It comes out exactly like the real thing! If you use a blender, it will taste as good, but will acquire more of a pudding texture.

Variations: Try a frozen mango/banana ice cream combination!

Add, after freezing, 1/4 cup raisins; or 3 T carob powder.

68

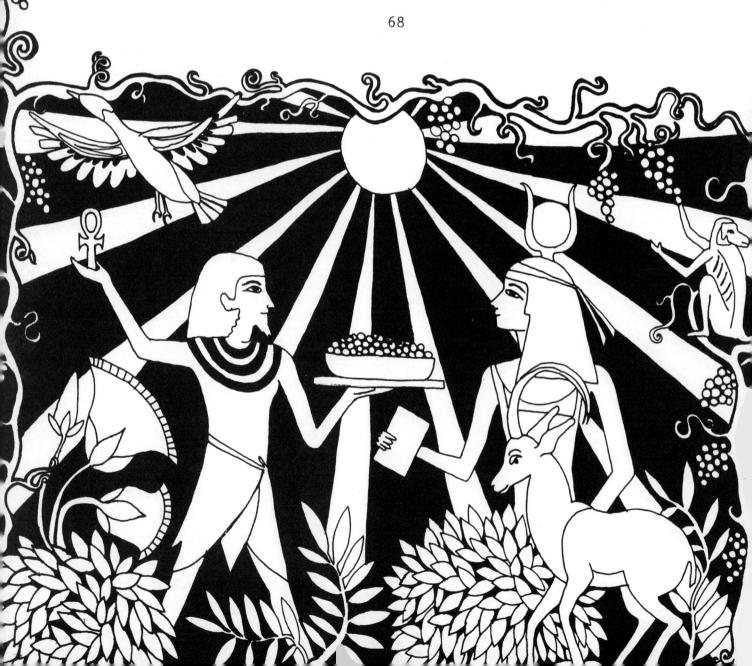

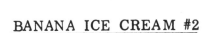

BANANA ICE CREAM #2

10 bananas   1 C soya powder   1/2 C tahini (8 T)

Blend the above ingredients and pour into individual containers. Place in freezer about 4-5 hours before serving. Makes about 1 1/2 quarts.

Variations: For Carobanana Ice Cream, proceed exactly as above, but add in 3 T
    carob powder. Try adding in a t of cloves with the carob for an exotic taste.
    For Almond Banana Ice Cream, add in 3 T of pure almond extract.
    For more of a vanilla taste, add in 3 T of freshly ground vanilla bean.
    You can vary this basic recipe endlessly: use orange and lemon peel,
Try homemade jams, and different fruit essences. Try different spices also.

69

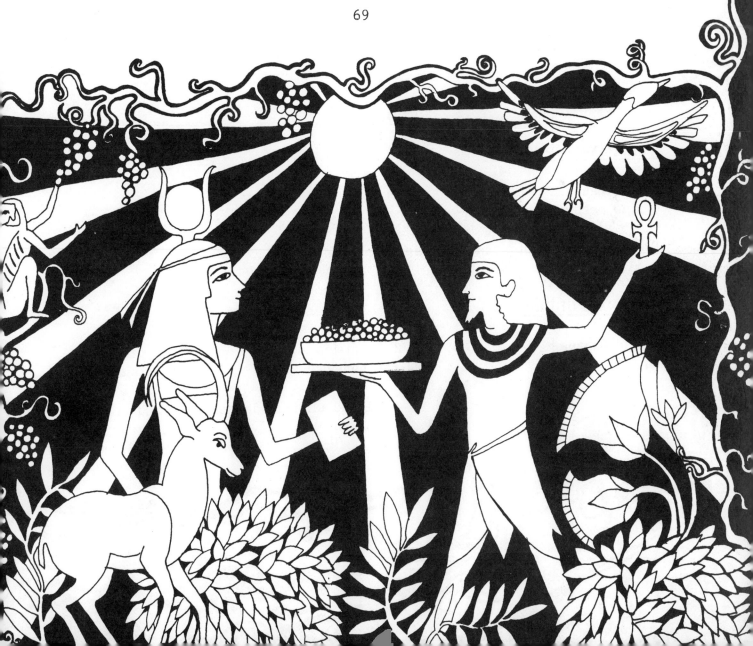

PEACH ICE CREAM

5 bananas
2 large peaches, chopped

1/2 C soya powder
4-5 T tahini

Blend all ingredients except for peaches. When smooth, add in peach chunks and freeze until served (at least 4 hours). Makes about 1 quart. For variety, use any kind of fresh fruit. Blueberries added to the above recipe are delicious.

PAPAYA SHERBERT

1/2 small papaya fruit
1/2 ripe banana
juice of 1 orange

1 slice pineapple
1/2 t vanilla extract
1 T honey

Cut up papaya, blend. Add other ingredients. Pour into freezer tray, and freeze until almost set. Remove and whip again in blender. Return to freezer for 2-3 hours. Makes about 1/2 quart.

PUDDINGS

PERSIMMON PUDDING

3 ripe bananas
4 ripe persimmons

1 T honey
1 t vanilla extract

Blend all ingredients, chill, and serve. For 4 - 6.

BANANA PUDDING

6 ripe bananas

1 1/2 C raisins
1 T raw honey

1/2 C apple juice
1/4 t nutmeg

Blend all ingredients, chill and serve. For 6 - 8.

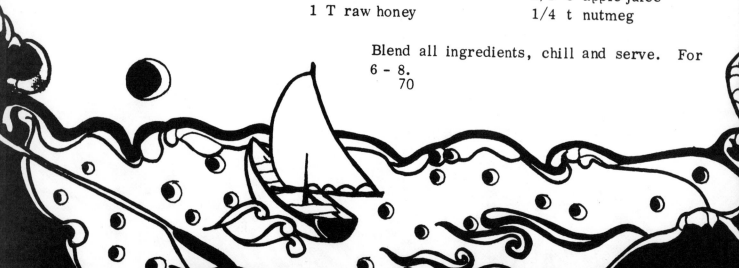

COCONUT-BANANA PUDDING

1 whole coconut
6 ripe bananas
1 T honey

1 T carob powder
1 t almond extract
1/4 t cloves or nutmeg

Use both the milk and meat from the coconut and blend. Add in the other ingredients, blending until smooth. Chill and serve in tall parfait glasses. Top with a few fresh berries and mint leaves. For 6 - 8.

Variations: Replace the bananas with another blended fruit, and leave out the coconut milk -- for example, coconut-blueberry. Or, leave out the coconut and blend the bananas with a fruit. Use cinnamon in place of the cloves or nutmeg.

APPLE NUT CREAM

3 apples (yellow delicious are good)
3/4 C cashews, soaked
3/4 C rejuvelac or water

2/3 C soya powder
1 T tahini

Chop the apples after coring, and blend all ingredients. Makes about 3 cups. Try any firm fruit and different kinds of nuts for variety.

PINEAPPLE SUNDAE

3 C crushed fresh pineapple
3 C grated apples
3 C apple nut cream (above)

6 T chopped pecans
6 fresh strawberries

Mix pineapple and grated apples. Fill up 12 ounce glasses with alternate layers of fresh fruit and apple nut cream. Sprinkle pecans on top of each glass, and place a strawberry in the center of each. For 6.

Variations: Use mangoes in place of the pineapples.
for a sub-acid - sweet combination. Or
try a strawberry-apple mixture. Other
replacements: apricots, cherries.

71

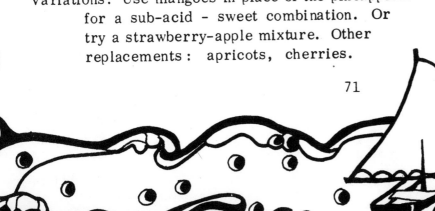

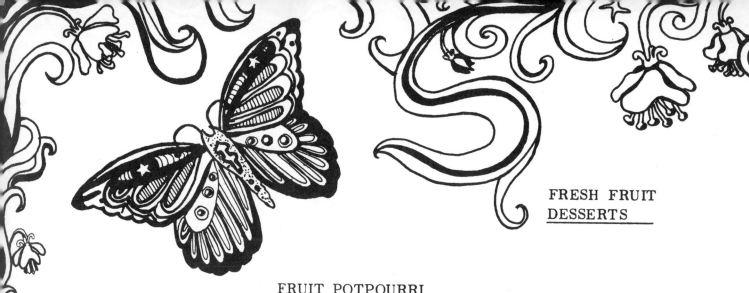

FRUIT POTPOURRI

4 apples
2 bananas
1/2 C raisins

4 pears
10 chopped dates
4 T freshly squeezed orange juice

Grate the apples and stir in orange juice. Slice the pears and bananas, add a little orange juice and mix with apples in a bowl. Add dates and raisins, stir together. For 4.

PINEAPPLE POTPOURRI

1/2 fresh pineapple

1/2 fresh coconut

Cut pineapple into chunks. Grate coconut or run through food grinder. Mix both together for a simple, exquisite and nutritious dessert. Coconut contains complete proteins; pineapple contains bromelain, a helpful digestive enzyme. Serves 4 - 6.

APPLE DELIGHT

2 apples, cored
1/2 C raisins, soaked
1 T lemon juice
1/2 t cinnamon

1/2 C sunflower seeds
1/2 C rejuvelac or
    spring water
4 T chopped walnuts

4 - 8 hours before serving, grind sunflower seeds and lightly ferment in rejuvelac by allowing them to sit, covered, in a quiet corner. Shred the apples; blend in soaked raisins with lemon juice and cinnamon. Fold in sunflower yoghurt, and serve in sherbert glasses. Top with chopped nuts. For 2. For a tarter flavor, ferment the seeds 12 hours.

72

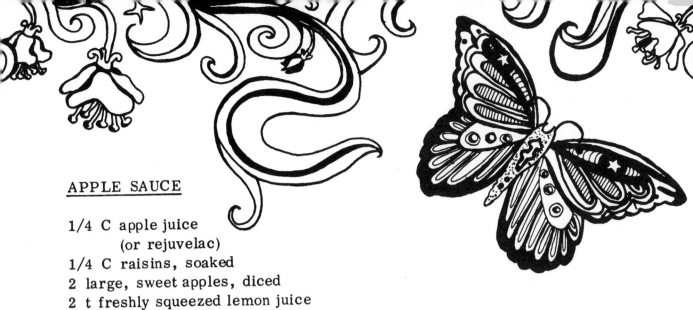

APPLE SAUCE

1/4 C apple juice
    (or rejuvelac)
1/4 C raisins, soaked
2 large, sweet apples, diced
2 t freshly squeezed lemon juice
1/2 t ginger

Pour the liquid into the blender. At a low speed, work in the raisins, followed with the apples and lemon juice. Blend in the ginger for a tang. This treat can be a complete meal. For 2.

APPLE GINGER TREAT

2 large, hard apples, grated
2-3 T freshly grated ginger root

Mix both these ingredients in a bowl and serve. It is refreshing and clean tasting. Try it! For 2.

APPLE BASKETS

4 large, tart red apples
1 C fresh pineapple, crushed
1 C seedless grapes
1/2 C raisins
8-10 T apple nut cream (see page 71)

Slice the apple tops off. Carefully core and scoop out about 2/3 of the pulp. Mix this with the other ingredients. Refill the baskets, and replace the top, or use some apple peel for a handle. For 4.

Variation: If nut cream is not available,
       blend 1/2 C of the fruit mixture
       together for a binder.

73

SLICED APPLE GOODIES

2 fresh red apples
8 T apple nut cream (see page 61)
8 T cashew (or any) nut butter

Core the apples and slice horizontally. Put together sandwich style with alternating layers of nut butter and nut cream. For 2.

Variations: Use any of the puddings outlined earlier in this chapter. Use other firm fruits: peaches, nectarines, pears.
For a variety of fillings, blend up fruit you have on hand with enough seed meal to attain a thick consistency. Nut butters will also help thicken the filling.

RAINBOW BANANA DESSERT

1 whole coconut, shredded <u>or</u>
4 C dried, shredded coconut

juices listed below
4 bananas

Divide the coconut onto 4 plates, and add one coloring to each plate.

red - 4 T beet juice
orange - 3 T carrot juice, 1 T beet juice
green - 4 T juiced greens - spinach, comfrey, celery
brown - 4 T carob powder moistened in 3-4 T water

The juice amounts above are for fresh coconut. Increase amounts for dried coconut. Slice bananas lengthwise and quarter horizontally. Roll each segment in a different combination of colored coconut. Arrange, rainbow-style, on a platter. For 4 - 6.

BANANA CANDLES

4 thick slices of fresh pineapple
2 bananas
1 C grapes (seedless)

2 brazil nuts
4 T chopped nuts

Core the pineapple slices. Cut bananas in half crosswise (not lengthwise). Place the banana's flat end in the middle of the cored pineapple, so that its pointed end is up. Cut the brazil nut in half, lengthwise, and sharpen one end with a knife. Insert the unsharpened end in the top of the banana. Garnish the pineapple with the chopped nuts and grapes.

When read to serve, light the brazil nut. It will burn for a few minutes because of its high oil content! Long straight bananas make the best candles. For 4.

BANAPPLE TREAT

2 apples, chopped
1 C raisins

1 banana
2 C spring water

Soak the raisins in warm water until soft (4 hours or more). Drain raisins and put on top of chopped apples. Slice banana over apples and raisins. Serve with the nut cream below. For 2 - 4.

ALMOND NUT BUTTER CREAM

1 C soak water (from recipe above)
1 C soaked almonds

2-4 T coconut oil
1 T honey, unfiltered

Soak almonds 4 hours or more. Put 2 T of oil in the blender. Add nuts and process until a crunchy or a smooth texture is reached. Add in a T of oil at a time, if needed. Blend in the honey and the soak water from the raisins. Makes about 1 1/2 cups.

NUT BUTTER STUFFED BANANAS

2 ripe bananas
1/4 C water or rejuvelac (approximately)

1 C nuts -- cashew-almond
2-4 T coconut oil

Soak nuts 4 hours. You can use any kind of nut, or any combination of nut and seed. Drain off water. Put 2 T of oil in the blender, and while the motor is running, slowly add the nuts. Process until you achieve a thick, buttery consistency. Add more oil if the butter becomes too thick. Different nuts have different amounts of oil in them, so the amount of oil you add to the blender will vary, depending on the type of nut you choose. Makes about 1 cup of nut butter.

Now, after making the nut butter, slice the bananas lengthwise. Spread the nut butter on both halves, and stick the halves together again. Take the remaining nut butter (hopefully about 1/2 cup) and blend with the same amount of water. Pour this nut butter cream over the stuffed bananas and serve to 2 - 4.

DIPPED STRAWBERRIES

1 C sunflower seed meal
1 C rejuvelac

1/2 papaya, peeled and cubed
1 pint fresh strawberries

Soak the seed in the rejuvelac 4 hours or more to make a yoghurt. Blend the yoghurt with the cubed papaya. Put this sauce in a serving bowl, and serve the berries in another bowl. Let your guests dip their own berries into the sauce. For 2 - 4. Use any other berry or any other cubed fruit.

DEAD FOODS produce
DYING BODIES

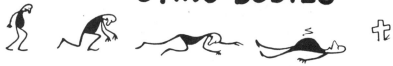

LIVE FOODS   **LIVE BODIES!**

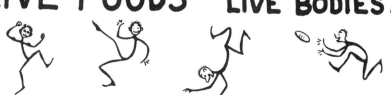

Vegetable Salad Creations

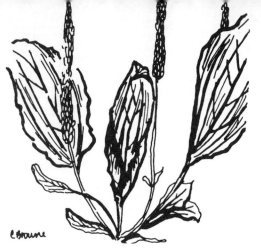

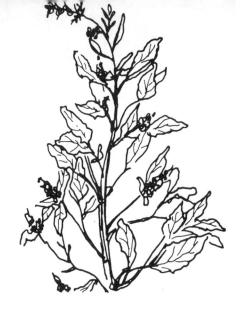

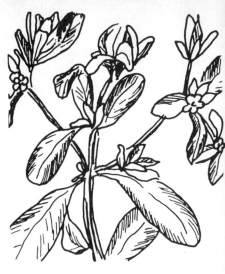

PLANTAIN— The young leaves are rich in vitamin A but not terribly exciting to eat. I like to make a chlorophyll broth by gathering the leaves of many greens—plantain, dandelion, nettles, wild lettuce, etc.

LAMBSQUARTERS— This common weed has a taste similar to spinach but is far more tasty and nutritious.

PURSLANE— This delightful sour-flavored pot herb has juicy leaves and flourishes as a weed in cultivated gardens. It is still grown in Europe and the Middle East as a vegetable.

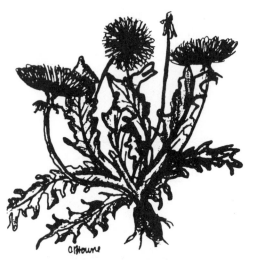

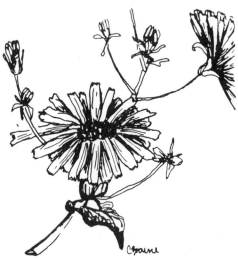

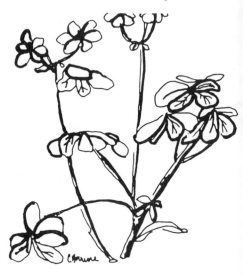

DANDELION AND CHICORY— The most important thing to consider in gathering these common plants is to harvest the leaves prior to blooming. Afterwards the plants take on a bitter taste. Young leaves are most tasty when finely chopped.

SORREL— This plant has a culinary reputation in France in famous sauces; it is splendid in salads and in vegetable dishes. Being related to rhubarb, it has a faintly similar tart flavor.

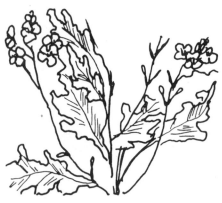

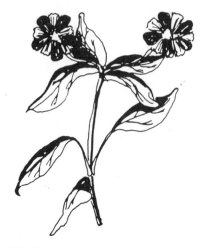

WILD MUSTARD— This plant has a pleasant tangy taste (provided you have already developed an affection for domestic mustard and collard greens).

COMMON MALLOW— Globe trotting mallows have been used as food for animals and man for centuries.

CHICKWEED— This peppery flavored plant is good.

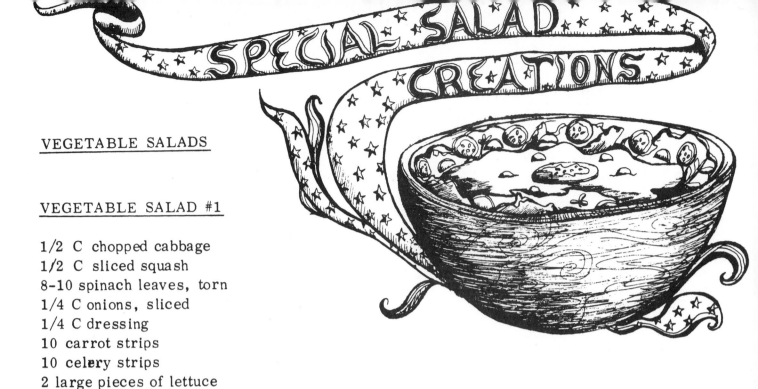

VEGETABLE SALADS

VEGETABLE SALAD #1

1/2 C chopped cabbage
1/2 C sliced squash
8-10 spinach leaves, torn
1/4 C onions, sliced
1/4 C dressing
10 carrot strips
10 celery strips
2 large pieces of lettuce

Line individual salad bowls with the pieces of lettuce. Mix together the cabbage, squash, spinach and onions; add the dressing to moisten. Place this in the lettuce-lined bowls. Garnish with the carrot strips and celery strips. (Try to take your celery strips from the top of the stalk. Slice thinly, and leave the celery leaves on.) For 2 - 4.

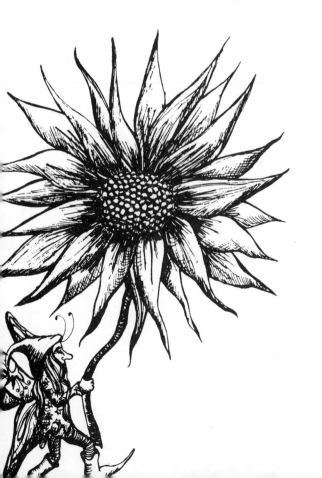

VEGETABLE SALAD #2

1 C grated carrots
1 C shredded cucumber
1 C pink sauerkraut (see page
3 C greens, torn into bite-size pieces

Prepare the vegetables independently, and arrange in three separate, small mounds on individual plates of shredded greens. Serve your favorite dressing separately. For 2 - 4.

BASIC VEGETABLE SALAD

1 C any type of green
1 C any vegetable -- grated, chopped
1 C any type of sprout
1/4-1/2 C seed sauce

Mix all together with love. For 2.

79

SOMETHING'S FISHY SALAD

2 C shredded parsnips

1 C finely sliced celery

1/2 C homemade mayonnaise (page 116)

1 T lemon juice

2 t finely minced green onion

3/4 t kelp

Mix parsnips, celery. Blend together the mayonnaise, lemon, onion, and kelp. Blend the parsnip-celery mixture with the sauce for just a few seconds, so that it becomes thick and heavy. Toss lightly and serve on greens. For 2 - 4.

SLIGHTLY SALMON SALAD

3 medium carrots, chopped or grated

1/2 C cashew nuts, chopped

1 T nut butter

1 T seed cheese

1 t rejuvelac or water

1/4 t kelp

1/8 t dill

Blend the carrots with the nuts, turning the blender on and off to push stray carrot pieces down under the blades. Blend in the other ingredients. Process this in batches if your blender gets filled up over the 2/3 mark. Blend until you have a thick, tuna-fishy texture. Serve on top of a bed of greens. For 2 - 4.

You can replace the nut butter with another T each of nut meal and oil. For a crunchy texture, mix in 1 cup of coarsely chopped fresh string beans. Grated squash will also work well.

CAULIFLOWER SALAD

1 very small head of cauliflower

6-8 leaves curly endive

4-5 bermuda onion slices

2 small stalks celery, sliced

1 T fresh chervil or 1/2 t dried

1 T fresh herbs (parsley, chives, thyme)

Break cauliflowerettes off into bite-size pieces. Chop the core into the salad as well. Break the endive into pieces, separate the onion slices into rings, and add the fresh herbs. Mix all. Add a dressing of your choice. For 4.

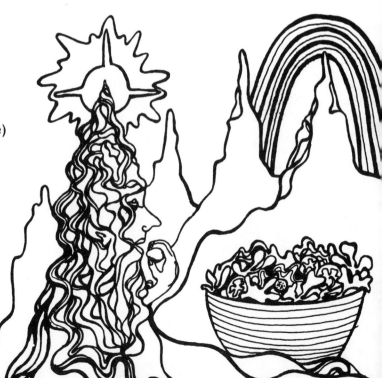

RED AND WHITE CAULIFLOWER SALAD

1/2 small head cauliflower
1 red pepper

2 tomatoes
1/8 t cayenne

Cut up cauliflower into thin slices and pieces. Dice pepper and tomatoes. Add all together. Serve with a seed sauce to keep the white effect. For 2 - 4.

Variation: Add in 4 T of finely minced parsley for green, or 1/2 cup shredded red cabbage for more color.

SWEET PEAS AND SPROUTS

1 C fresh sweet peas
1 C mung bean sprouts
1/2 C shredded red leaf lettuce

1/4 C shredded summer squash
1 t freshly chopped dill
6 romaine lettuce leaves

Mix all together except the romaine lettuce. Use avocado mayonnaise, page 127, to bind all the ingredients together. Serve on top of the romaine lettuce. For 2 - 4.

RAW GOULASH

2-3 ears of fresh corn
1 C diced tomatoes

1 C shredded squash
1/4 C chopped green onion
1/4 C chopped bell pepper
pinch of thyme
pinch of marjoram

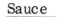
Sauce
1 tomato
4 T sunflower seed meal
1/8 t cayenne pepper
juice of 1/2 lemon

Scrape the corn off the cob. Use the back of the knife to press all the juice out of the cob. Mix all the ingredients together, and serve in a lettuce leaf lined bowl. Pour the sauce over the goulash before serving. For 4.

81

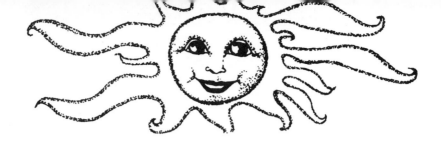

CUCUMBER SALAD

2 large sliced cucumbers (unpeeled)
3 large tomatoes, cubed
1 red pepper, finely chopped
1/2 C sliced celery

juice of 1/4 lemon
2 T freshly chopped chives
1 clove pressed garlic
2 t kelp

Mix the cucumbers and tomatoes together in the serving bowl. Blend all the other ingredients together for a sauce, and pour over the tomatoes and cucumbers just before serving. For 6 - 8.

CUCUMBER-RADISH SALAD

2 organic cucumbers
8-12 radishes
1/2 medium-size onion
2 tomatoes, diced

1 C indoor greens
2 T lemon juice
2 T coconut oil
2 t kelp

Slice cucumbers, leaving the skins on. Slice radishes and onion very finely. If you use greens other than indoor greens, tear them into bite size pieces. Put all ingredients in a bowl, and pour the oil over it. Toss lightly. Mix the kelp and lemon juice; pour it over the salad and toss again before serving. For 6.

Variations: Use fresh wild edibles for greens: comfrey, sorrel, lambsquarters, dandelion, chicory. Add in a few peppermint leaves for a cool, refreshing taste. Try a pinch of fresh dill, too.

BROCCOLI SALAD

1 1/2 C broccoli, thinly sliced
1 1/2 C shredded red cabbage

1 C sauerkraut
1/4 C minced onion

Mix all ingredients together. Serve with a fermented seed sauce. For 2 - 4.

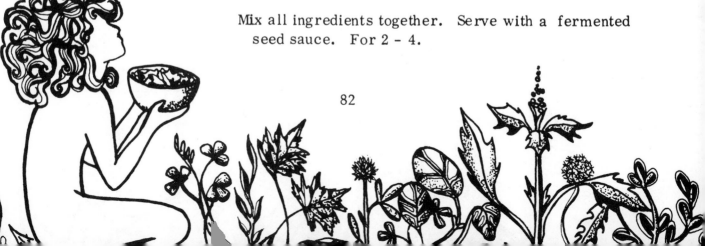

82

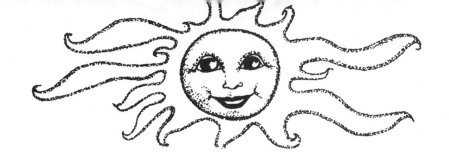

GUACAMOLE SALAD

1 ripe avocado
1 lemon, juiced
2 tomatoes, finely diced

1/2 red pepper
1 T spanish onion, minced
1 t kelp

Using a fork, blend the avocado to a creamy consistency. Mash in the lemon juice and kelp. Mix in the other ingredients. This is a good side dish salad. For 2 - 4.

CORN SALAD

2 ears fresh corn
2 tomatoes, chopped

1/2 cucumber, sliced
2 C alfalfa sprouts

Slice the corn off the cob. Put sprouts in a serving bowl, and lay the corn kernels in the middle of the sprout bed. Surround the corn with the bright red tomatoes. Then place all the cucumber slices around the outer edge of the bowl. For 2.

Variation: Add 1/2 cup each of red pepper and sliced celery. Add a pinch of cayenne.

ROOT VEGETABLES

ROOT VEGETABLE SALAD

1/2 C carrots, shredded
1/2 C parsnips, shredded
2 T onions, minced

1/4 C fermented seed sauce
pinch of cayenne
1 1/2 C greens

Mix column 1 ingredients together with the seed sauce and cayenne. Serve on top of a bed of greens in individual salad bowls.   For 2.

83

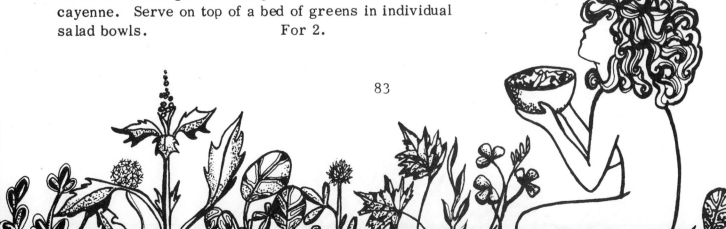

LOVEL'S EARTHY SALAD

1 large beet, grated   2-3 stalks celery, grated
2 carrots, grated   6-8 large comfrey leaves

Leave all skins on vegetables, scrub well before grating. Mix all vegetables
together. Enjoy with a light vegetable dressing. For 2 - 4.

COLE SLAW

1 C grated rutabaga   1 C carrots, grated
1 C grated green cabbage

Mix well and serve with avocado mayonnaise, page 127. For 2.

Variation: Use this as a stuffing for 2 hollowed out bell peppers.

ROOT SALAD #1

1 C grated parsnips   1 C grated turnip
1 C grated squash   1 C grated potato
1/4 C minced leeks   1/4 green pepper, minced

Scrub the vegetables well, and leave their coats on, since the majority of
their vitamins are in or near the skin. Toss all ingredients together and
serve over a bed of greens or sprouts. Or enjoy as is for a hearty salad.

84

ROOT SALAD #2

1 C grated beets
1 C grated potatoes
1 C grated Jerusalem artichokes
1/2 C grated radishes
2 t kelp

Scrub all vegetables well
before mixing. 2 - 4.

RED COMMUNAL SALAD

2 C finely grated beets   4 T coconut oil
4 T green onion, minced   1 lemon, squeezed

Mix all together thoroughly.   For 2.

Variations: Add in 1 small grated potato, or a turnip or parsnip. Jerusalem
          artichoke or kohlrabi would also blend well. Try any root vege-
          table -- they all combine well together.

BEET FREAK SALAD

3 medium beets   1 T tamari
2 stalks celery   1 T lime juice
2 T coconut oil   1 t mixed spices

Shred or grate the beets and celery.   Experiment with different shredded
textures to see which you prefer. A more coarsely grated salad will offer
more chewing.

Take 2/3 cup of the mixed shredded vegetables. Put in blender with all
the other ingredients and process until smooth. Pour the sauce over the
beets and celery. Let it stand about an hour before serving. For 2 - 4.

TURNIP SALAD

2 C grated turnip
2 Jerusalem artichokes, grated
1/2 C sliced leeks
6-8 comfrey leaves
1 T dulse

Tear comfrey into bite-size
pieces, and mix with all
the other ingredients.
Sprinkle the dry dulse
over the top of the
salad. For 2 - 4.

85

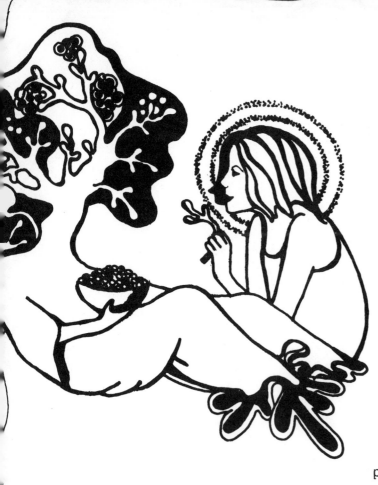

TOSSED GREEN SALAD

  2 C romaine, endive, chicory, or lettuce
  1/4 C parsley, minced
  1/4 C chives, minced
   1/4 C watercress leaves
   1/4 C green onions, minced
  1/2 lemon, juiced
  2 T coconut oil
  1 T nut meal

Cut the greens into bite sized pieces. Use the greens in any combination: if you have all on hand, put in 1/4 cup of each. Add the finely chopped parsley, chives, watercress and onions. Into a small jar, place the lemon juice and oil. Shake well and pour over the greens so that each leaf is well coated. Sprinkle the nut meal over all. For 2.

DANDELION SALAD

10-12 dandelion leaves
1 C alfalfa sprouts

1 tomato
1 leek

Make a bed of the alfalfa sprouts. Tear the dandelion leaves into edible pieces. Slice the tomato and the white portion of the leek over all the greens. For 2. Use the dandelions you find growing in the ground about you, and wash them well.

Variations: Use nay type of wild green edible you find growing about you: chicory, sorrel, purslane, chickweed, persimmon, comfrey, burdock, etc. If you have a choice, pick the younger, more tender leaves.

LAMBSQUARTER AND DANDELION SALAD

1 C fresh lambsquarter leaves
2 C tender dandelion leaves
3/4 C alfalfa sprouts
1/3 C sunflower seeds, soaked
1/3 C coconut oil

3 T lemon juice
1/2 t crushed garlic
1/4 t paprika
1/4 t kelp (or more, according to taste)

Toss together the first group of live foods. Sprinkle the second group of ingredients on top of that. For 2 - 4.

Variation: Any kind of wild edible would be tasty in place of the lambsquarter or dandelion leaves. There are many informative books out on "eating the weeds." Find them at your health food store.

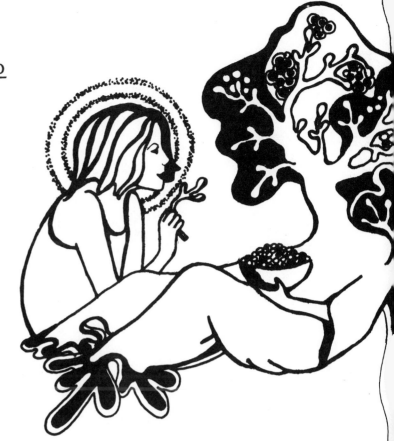

MUSHROOMS AND GREENS

4-6 spinach leaves
4-6 beet greens
1 C sliced mushrooms

1/4 C green onions, chopped
1 t kelp

Lay greens down in a serving bowl; spread mushrooms around edge. Sprinkle onions, kelp, and garlic in center. Let your diners see and enjoy this salad before tossing.

Variation: Any kind of dark, chlorophyll-rich green would be delicious with the mushrooms: watercress-mushroom is an excellent combination. Try wild edibles as well.

87

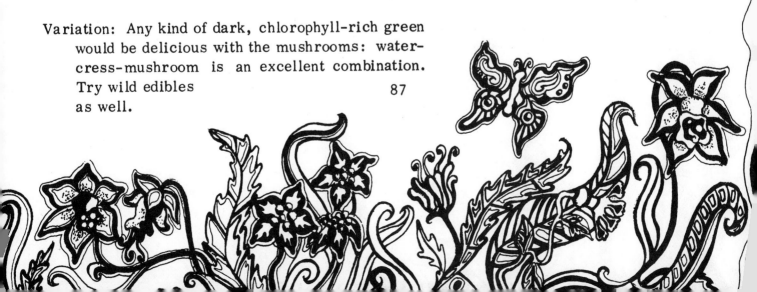

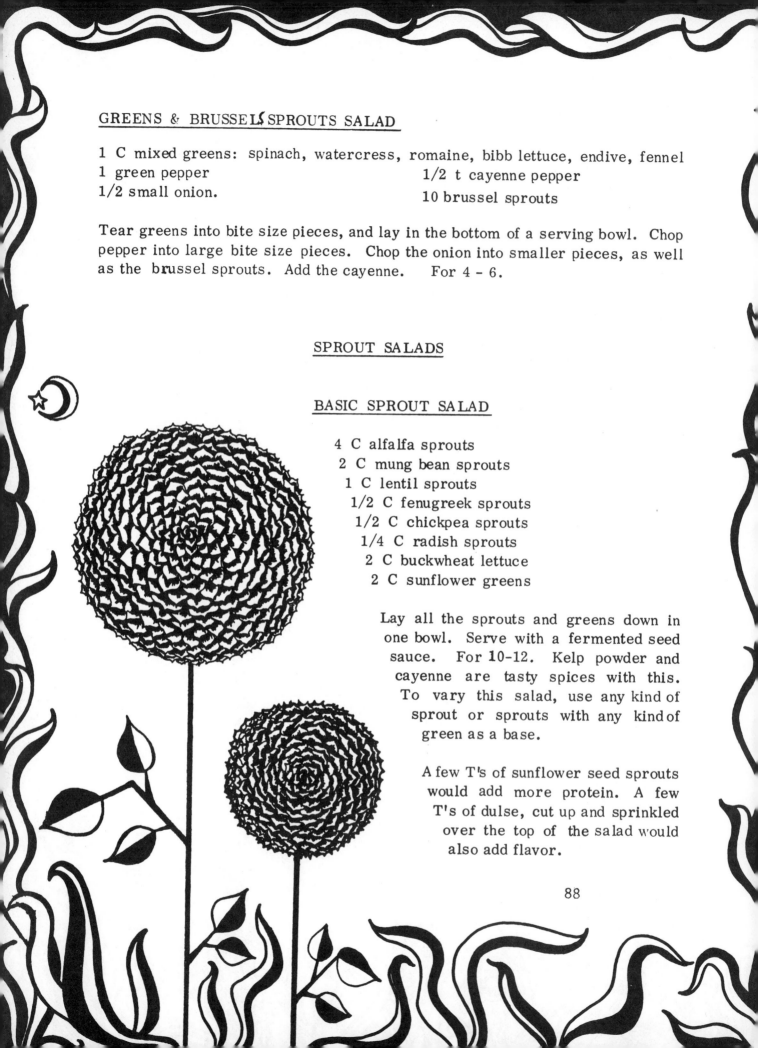

GREENS & BRUSSELS SPROUTS SALAD

1 C mixed greens: spinach, watercress, romaine, bibb lettuce, endive, fennel
1 green pepper   1/2 t cayenne pepper
1/2 small onion.   10 brussel sprouts

Tear greens into bite size pieces, and lay in the bottom of a serving bowl. Chop pepper into large bite size pieces. Chop the onion into smaller pieces, as well as the brussel sprouts. Add the cayenne. For 4 - 6.

SPROUT SALADS

BASIC SPROUT SALAD

4 C alfalfa sprouts
2 C mung bean sprouts
1 C lentil sprouts
1/2 C fenugreek sprouts
1/2 C chickpea sprouts
1/4 C radish sprouts
2 C buckwheat lettuce
2 C sunflower greens

Lay all the sprouts and greens down in one bowl. Serve with a fermented seed sauce. For 10-12. Kelp powder and cayenne are tasty spices with this. To vary this salad, use any kind of sprout or sprouts with any kind of green as a base.

A few T's of sunflower seed sprouts would add more protein. A few T's of dulse, cut up and sprinkled over the top of the salad would also add flavor.

88

KOREAN BEAN SPROUT SALAD

4 C fresh bean sprouts (mung, lentil)
2 T finely chopped green onions
5 T coconut oil

4 T tamari
1/2 clove garlic, chopped
1 t kelp

Combine all ingredients. Serves 6 – 8. Any kind of sprout will combine well.

HIPPOCRATES LUNCHEON SALAD

2 C alfalfa sprouts
2 C buckwheat lettuce
1 C mung bean sprouts
1/2 C fenugreek sprouts

1/2 C sunflower seed sprouts
1/2 C zucchini
1 red pepper, chopped
1 T kelp

Place all in a large salad bowl, and serve with a
fermented seed sauce. For 6 – 8.

When serving a greater number of diners, you
can let each person create his or her own
salad by putting each ingredient on the table
in its own serving dish. Each individual
will choose that which is most appealing.
You can vary infinitely what you place in
front of your diners -- any fresh vegetable, cut or sliced, diced or minced.
In effect, you will be creating your
own salad bar.

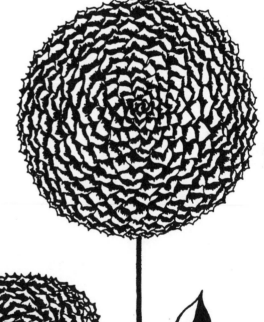

Some vegetable ideas:
- peppers cut in rings
- onions, sliced in rings
- freshly cut chives
- shredded red cabbage
- shredded beets, turnips
- shredded mustard greens
- favorite weeds
- tomatoes, cut in wedges
- diced avocado

89

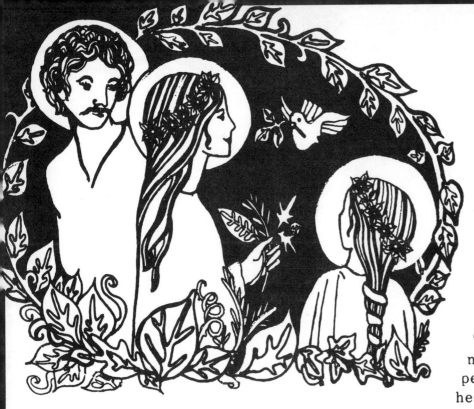

LENTIL SALAD

1 C lentil sprouts
4 scallions, chopped
2 stalks celery, chopped
1/2 green pepper, sliced
6-8 comfrey leaves, torn
1 t kelp

Combine all ingredients and serve with a sunflower seed sauce. For 2 - 4.

To serve a larger group, add one more cup of lentil sprouts. Chick-pea sprouts will add more of a heavy, crunchy texture.

MIXED ALFALFA SALAD

2 C alfalfa sprouts
2 C mixed greens:
    chicory, bibb lettuce,
    red leaf lettuce, spinach,
    kale, sunflower greens,
    buckwheat lettuce

1/2 C radishes, finely sliced or
1/2 C radish sprouts
1/2 C celery, diced
8-10 pepper rings (red or green)
2-3 T sesame seed meal
1 T kelp

Make a bed of the mixed greens in a serving bowl, and put the alfalfa sprouts on top. Decorate the bowl with the other ingredients. For 4 - 6. Use a fermented seed sauce with this for a complete meal salad. Homemade sauerkraut will complement this salad well. Mix it in with the greens, place it around the outer edge of the bowl or serve it separately as a side dish.

ALFALFA-AVOCADO SALAD

3 C alfalfa sprouts
1 avocado
1 tomato

1 stalk celery
2-4 T minced onion
1 t each: cayenne pepper, kelp

Mash the avocado with a fork, and chop the tomato. Put both in blender and process for 4-5 seconds, just until both are mixed together. Put the other ingredients in a serving bowl and pour the sauce over all. Enjoy! For 2 - 4.

Variations: Instead of blending, cube the avocado and tomato, and use a different sauce to dress the salad.

SIMPLE SPROUT SALAD

2 C favorite sprouts
    (alfalfa, mung)
2 T coconut oil
1/2 t kelp
few bits dulse

Mix all together, and eat any
time. For 1. This will be a
nutritious pick-up snack.

COMPLETE PROTEIN
SALAD SNACK

1 C wheat sprouts
1 C chick pea sprouts
2 T minced parsley
1 t vegetable seasoning
1 t kelp
3 T coconut oil
1 T lemon juice.

Mix the sprouts together with the minced parsley and seasonings. Pour the liquids
over all. Take it to work. For 1.

SWEET WHEAT

1 C sprouted wheat
2 T ground sesame seed
1 t vegetable seasoning (optional)

1 t kelp
2 T fermented seed sauce

Mix all together for a hearty salad or side dish. This will make a good portable snack
as well. For 1 or 2. See the taboule recipe, page 33, for more wheat sprout ideas.

WHEAT SPROUT SALAD

2 C fresh wheat sprouts
1/2 C grated carrots
1 small onion, minced
3 T coconut oil

1 T lemon juice
1 t kelp
3 T unhulled sesame seeds
2 lettuce leaves

Mix sprouts, carrots and onions with the oil and lemon juice. Sprinkle with kelp,
garnish with sesame seeds. Fill lettuce cups or mound on a bed of sprouts. For 2.

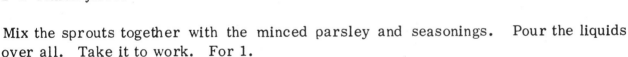

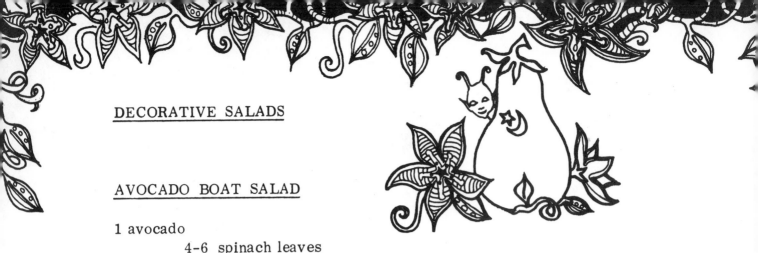

DECORATIVE SALADS

AVOCADO BOAT SALAD

1 avocado
    4-6 spinach leaves
        3 T each:
               shredded carrot, minced onion, minced celery
               2 T coconut oil
               1 t freshly squeezed lemon juice

Place half a peeled avocado on a bed made of the spinach leaves. Mix the chopped vegetables with the oil and lemon. Pile this into the center of the avocado and serve. For 2.

When this is to be the main course, allow 1 whole avocado per person, and use more of the vegetable mixture. Any kind of shredded vegetable would be fine: try carrot-celery-beet; parsley-beet-cucumber-carrot; lentil sprouts-tomato-pepper-onion.

CUCUMBER BOATS

1 small cucumber
4 lettuce leaves <u>or</u>
1 C salad greens
2 T coconut oil
1 t tamari

2 T grated parsnips or beets
2 T homemade pink sauerkraut
1 T celery, shredded
1 T carrots, grated
1 T minced parsley

Peel the cucumbers if they have been waxed or sprayed (try to get organic cucumbers for this salad). Cut them in half lengthwise and hollow out the centers. Place the boats on top of the greens. Mix the chopped vegetables together with the chopped cucumber hearts. Moisten with the oil and tamari, and fill the cucumber boats with this mixture. For a sail, glue a triangular piece of paper onto a toothpick, and stick the toothpick sail into the salad. For 2.

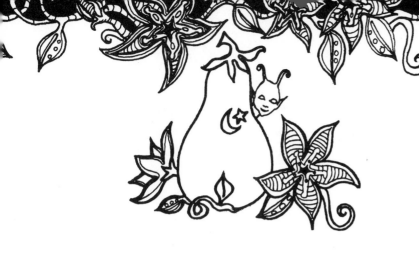

TOMATO ROSE SALAD

3-4 spinach leaves
1 tomato
2-3 T celery
1 T onion, minced
1 T favorite dressing

On an individual serving plate, make a bed of the spinach leaves. For each serving, cut a large, juicy, ripe tomato (unpeeled) almost all the way through, into six petal-like sections. Arrange like a rose on the bed of greens. In the center place the minced celery and onion, cover with the dressing. For 1 rose.

NUTTY TOMATO BOWLS

2 large, ripe tomatoes
2 T mashed avocado
2 T minced parsley
2 T minced celery

2 T chopped pecans
4-6 bibb lettuce leaves <u>or</u>
2 C alfalfa sprouts

Cut the top lid off from the tomatoes. Scoop out the pulp and drain off the juice. Put the pulp and juice in a bowl and mix with the avocado, parsley and celery. Fill the tomato bowls with the mixture. Top with a T of the chopped pecans, and place on top of the lettuce leaves, or use the sprouts as a bed. For 2 bowls.

For more flavor, mash a pinch of cayenne and kelp into the avocado. Radish sprouts also add zest.

GUACAMOLE STUFFED TOMATOES FOR TWO

Guacamole Salad, page 151   2 large, ripe tomatoes

Hollow out the tomatoes as described above. Use the tomato pulp and juice in place of the diced tomatoes called for in the Guacamole Salad. Stuff the tomato bowls with the mixture.

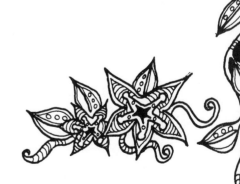

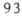

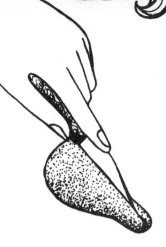

RAINBOW SALAD

1 C grated beet
  1 C grated carrot
    1 C grated white cabbage
      1 C grated red cabbage

1/2 C grated turnip
1/2 C grated parsnip
4-6 C dark greens: comfrey, beet
      greens, dandelion, chicory,
      buckwheat, sunflower greens

Keep the vegetables separate as you grate them. Arrange all in rainbow curves on a bed of the greens. For 6 - 8.

CHRISTMAS DAY SALAD

2 C beet greens
2 C spinach leaves

2 C comfrey leaves
3 C shredded beets
1 T coconut oil

Tear the greens into edible pieces, and mix them with the oil. Put in a clear bowl, and put the beets on top. Incredible! For six.

VEGETABLE SALAD BOWL

1 small clove garlic
12-14 spinach leaves, torn
1/2 small head romaine lettuce, torn
1 small bunch watercress, separated
1 small bunch parsley, minced
3 stalks celery, sliced
1/4 medium onion, sliced into rings
1 scallion, chopped

1 small cucumber, sliced
1/2 small head cauliflower, chopped
6-8 sliced radishes
3 tomatoes, sliced
1 small green pepper, sliced
1 carrot, shredded
1 small summer, squash, sliced
1 ear corn, cut off cob

Cut the garlic clove and rub it over the inside of a large wooden serving bowl. Prepare all the greens and vegetables, and toss together. For 8 -10.

For a garnish, top this salad with 4-6 T of sesame seeds. To further vary this salad, try to make sure that the vegetables are cut into different sizes and shapes. Offer your diners a selection of dressings to choose from. Add in any other fresh vegetable if you do not find the ones listed here.

Sprouts to add:
    4 C alfalfa sprouts
    2 C mung sprouts
    2 C lentil sprouts

1 C chick pea sprouts
1/2 C radish sprouts

By adding these sprouts, you will be able to serve 14 - 16.

PLATTER VEGETABLE SALAD

4 C mixed salad greens
4 C sprouts
8-10 celery strips
8-10 cucumber strips
8-10 carrot sticks
8-10 tomato slices
8-10 onion rings
8-10 pepper rings
1/2 C chick pea sprouts

Dressing Ingredients
1/2 C sesame seeds
1/2 C minced parsley
2 T basil
2 T kelp
2 T dried dulse
1 C coconut oil
1 C safflower oil
1/2 C freshly squeezed lemon juice

In the center of a large platter, place the greens. (Use buckwheat lettuce, sunflower greens, watercress, beet greens, turnip greens, kale, chard, bok choy, dandelion leaves -- in any combination.) Surround the greens with the sprouts (alfalfa-mung-lentil-fenugreek). Then surround the sprouts with mounds of the other colorful vegetables. (Use the ones listed, or vegetables of your own choosing). Make an eye-pleasing, beautiful-to-behold platter. Let each diner select and combine the salad of his or her own choosing. For 4 - 6.

You can also set out the dressing ingredients separately, so each can make an individual dressing as well.

For larger numbers of guests, make up individual bowls of ingredients. Decorate each bowl with a contrasting-colored vegetable. See the listing of vegetables in the back of this book for additional vegetable ideas, or better yet, see what the fresh vegetable section of your natural foods store or grocery store has to offer.

SPROUT LOAF

1/2 cup each -- sunflower, radish, fenugreek,
   (of any three) lentil, and chickpea sprouts
1/2 cup each -- chopped celery, scallions,
   red and green pepper
tamari and kelp, to taste
basil to taste

Mix in enough seed cheese (of your choice), with all ingredients
to form a loaf.

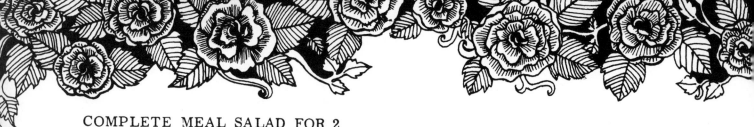

COMPLETE MEAL SALAD FOR 2

1 C alfalfa sprouts
1/2 C lentil sprouts
1/4 C mung sprouts
1/4 C fenugreek sprouts

1/2 C buckwheat lettuce
1/2 C sunflower greens

1/2 C parsnips or turnips, grated
1/2 C grated black radish

1/2 C red cabbage, sliced

1 tomato, sliced
1/2 avocado, sliced

In a salad bowl, make a bed out of the sprouts and greens. Arrange grated parsnips and black radish (white in color) around outer edge of bowl, on top of greens. Place red cabbage in center, circle with slices of red tomato and green avocado. Feast with your eyes! Serve with a seed sauce for additional complete proteins. For 2.

COMPLETE MEAL SALAD FOR 4

1 C alfalfa sprouts
1 C mung sprouts
1/2 C fenugreek sprouts
1/2 C sunflower sprouts

1 C buckwheat lettuce
1 C sunflower greens
1 C beet greens, chopped

1 small onion, minced
2 tomatoes, sliced
1 small zucchini, sliced
1/2 small cucumber, sliced
1 medium beet, grated
1 medium carrot, grated
2 stalks celery, sliced
1 T kelp

Mix sprouts and greens, place in a bowl, arrange vegetables decoratively on top.

COMPLETE MEAL SALAD FOR 4

1 1/2 C sunflower greens
1 1/2 C buckwheat lettuce

1 C mung sprouts
1 C alfalfa sprouts
1/2 C chick pea sprouts
1/8 C radish sprouts

4 sticks seed cheese stuffed celery
4 slices seed cheese stuffed pepper

2 small ears of tender fresh corn
8-12 cauliflowerettes
2 sliced rutabagas
1 sliced avocado

Make a bed of the greens, and arrange all vegetables attractively. Break the ears of corn in two, and let guests eat with their hands, or slice off cob. Serve with a fermented seed sauce.

FRUIT SALADS

SUB-ACID   SWEET FRUIT SALADS

FRUIT SALAD #1

3 apples, diced
2 pears, diced
2 bananas, sliced

2 C grapes
1/2 C shredded coconut

Mix all fruits together, and top with shredded coconut.   Add a sub-acid - sweet sauce, page 143. For variety, instead of dicing the apples and pears, shred them. The different texture makes it a different salad. For 4 - 6.

GRAPE/FRUIT SALAD

4 C grapes - green, red, purple
1 apple, shredded
1 nectarine, diced

1 banana, sliced
1/2 C currants

Cut grapes in half and de-seed. Cut up the rest of the fruit. Toss the ingredients. Garnish with currants. For 4 - 6.

SPRING SALAD

1 peach
1 apricot

8-10 cherries, pitted
1 nectarine

Slice these colorful fresh fruits. Arrange in a glass bowl so their gentle colors stand out.   For 2. This is tasty with the Cashew Apple Cream, page 71.

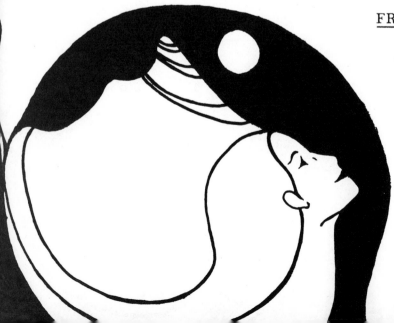

FRUIT TREAT

4 bananas, sliced
2 1/2 C green grapes
4 nectarines, sliced
2 juicy peaches, sliced
2 juicy pears, sliced
4 T coconut
1 C raisins, soaked (optional)

Mix all together. For a sauce, blend 2 cups of the mixed fruit with the soaked raisins, and drizzle over all. Top with coconut. For 4.

BLUEBERRY APPLE PEACH TREAT

2 apples, grated   1 C blueberries   2 peaches, sliced

Mix all together. You can enjoy this as is, or topped with a light sauce. See page 143. for Blueberry-Avocado Cream. For 2 - 4.

PERSIMMON SALAD

1 persimmon, sliced   2 C Tokay grapes, halved and seeded

Arrange slices of persimmon around a mound of the grapes. They are in season together and blend deliciously. For 2.

BASIC SUB-ACID - SWEET FRUIT SALAD

See the list of sub-acid and sweet fruits in the back of the book, and pick 3 or 4. See which your local farmer's market, natural food store, or supermarket carries, and which are ripe. Slice, dice, shred or chop the fruit up. You can top your fruit salad with a sauce, or enjoy it plain. See the sauce ideas on page 143 or make your own sauce by blending up a bit of your salad with some water or rejuvelac. Add sweetness by blending up a handful of soaked raisins or dates. A bowl full of fresh fruit, served chilled and untouched except for washing makes a beautiful salad too.

APPLE SALADS

APPLE WALDORF

4 red, ripe apples, chopped
1 C walnuts, well chopped

Apple Waldorf Dressing
1 C walnuts, well chopped
4-6 T rejuvelac or water
2-4 T coconut oil
1 T unfiltered honey (optional)

Blend the dressing until smooth. Put apples and nuts in attractive serving bowl, and pour the dressing over them. Top with a few more nuts. For 4.

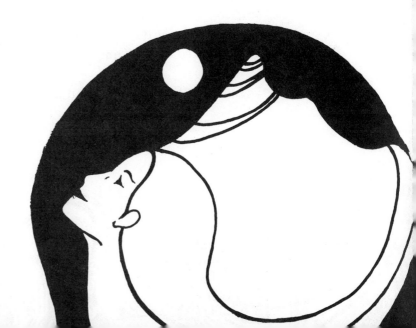

99

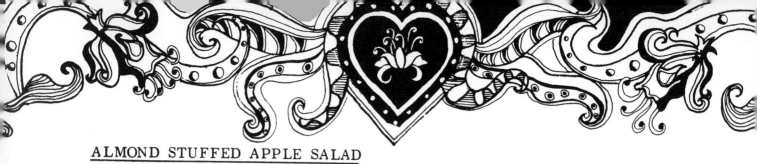

ALMOND STUFFED APPLE SALAD

2 large red, ripe apples
1 t fresh lemon juice
1/2 C almonds, ground or well chopped
1/2 C water or rejuvelac

1/4 t freshly grated ginger root
1/8 t cinnamon
2 circular pepper rings (large enough
      to fit over the apples)
4 slivered pecans

Quarter apples vertically and cut out the center seeds and pulp. Then cut away more pulp to leave about 3/8" of outer shell. Mash the pulp with the lemon juice.

Blend the almonds with the rejuvelac. Mix this unfermented seed cheese into the apple pulp.

Now, hold 3 sections of the apple together in your hand and fill with the apple-almond mixture. Fit the 4th section of the apple shell into place, and slide the green pepper collar over the whole shell.

Place the stuffed apple on leaves of green lettuce, and top with a few more spoonfuls of the center mixture and the pecans.

To eat, remove the collar, and let the apple sections fall open into an open flower design.

APPLE-DATE SALAD

2 apples, chopped
2 C red grapes, seeded
2 pears, cubed

4 T pineapple or apple juice
4 T pitted dates, soaked and chopped
2 T coconut, shredded

Combine first three fruits with the apple juice. Place in individual bowls and top with chopped, soaked dates, and coconut. For 2 - 4.

Variation: Leave out the grapes and pears, and enjoy just the
      apples and dates.

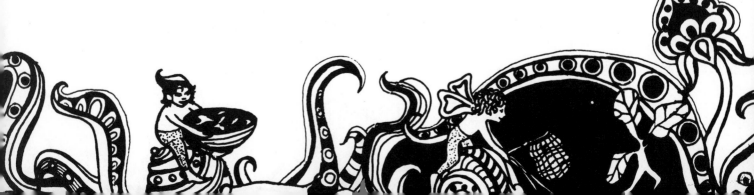

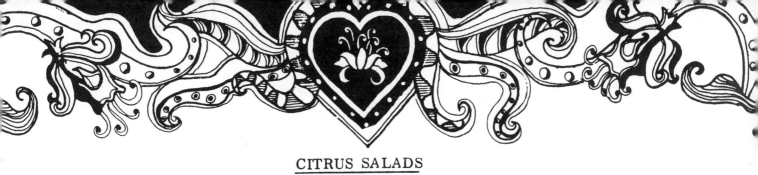

CITRUS SALADS

SLICED ORANGE SALAD

4 oranges   2 T coconut, grated

Slice the oranges, and sprinkle with freshly grated coconut. Delicious! For 2.

To slice oranges that have seeds, first peel. While holding the orange in your hand, use a serrated knife to cut the orange segments out of the orange core. This way, you leave the seeds in the core.

Grapefruit may be done the same way or one may take the segments apart and use scissors to open each segment along the top side. Press the seeds out, and if the little fibrous envelope seems too tough to use, remove the pulp completely.

MIXED FRUITS SALAD

2 oranges, sliced   3 C fresh pineapple chunks
1 grapefruit, sliced   2 C red and black grapes, pitted

Mix all fruits. Serve with Cashew Apple or Avocado Cream, page 144. For 4.

HEAVENLY CITRUS

3 oranges, sliced   1 C fresh grapefruit juice
2 tangerines, segmented   1 avocado, mashed

Mix grapefruit juice with the avocado; pour over oranges and tangerines. For 2.

> Variation: Make the sauce with orange/lemon juice instead of
> grapefruit juice. Use any type of ripe citrus fruit.

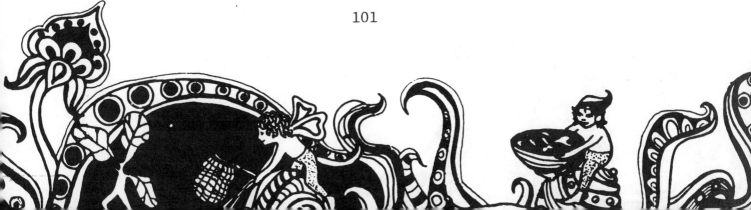

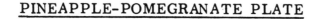

PINEAPPLE-POMEGRANATE PLATE

1 pomegranate, very ripe   2 C fresh pineapple chunks, crushed

Cut pomegranate in half and scoop out seeds to mix with the pineapple. Fill wine glasses with the mixture, or layer the glasses first with pomegranate, then pineapple. For 2.

PINEAPPLE & BERRIES

1/2 of a small pineapple   1 C blueberries
1 C strawberries   1 C blackberries
1 C raspberries

Make chunks with the pineapple and toss with the berries. For 6 - 8. If you desire a sauce, Avocado Cream, page 144, combines well.

PINEAPPLE-PAPAYA SALAD

1 large, ripe papaya   1 avocado, peeled and cubed
1 C fresh pineapple, diced   4-6 red leaf lettuce leaves
1 C fresh green grapes

De-seed papaya, saving seeds for a dressing. Cut peeled papaya in half, lengthwise, and lay each half on top of the red leaf lettuce. Mix the remaining fruits together, and spoon into the papaya halves. Top with a few T's of nut cream. For 2.

PINEAPPLE TREAT SALAD

1 C pineapple, cut into small chunks   1 apple, diced
2 oranges, cut up   1/2 C dates, chopped

Mix fruits together. Serve on individual plates and sprinkle dates over top. For 2.

PURE AND SIMPLE PINEAPPLE SALAD

3/4 C freshly grated coconut
2 C fresh pineapple chunks

102   Mix these two ingredients together. For 2.

PINEAPPLE SALAD DELUXE

1/2 of a pineapple
2-3 oranges
1 large grapefruit
1 C strawberries
2 tangerines, sectioned

Cut the pineapple into chunks, saving the shell. Cut out the orange and grapefruit meat. Place all the mixed fruits in the pineapple shell, and serve well chilled. For 4 - 6.

Variation: Add 1 cup of fresh coconut to the mixed fruits.

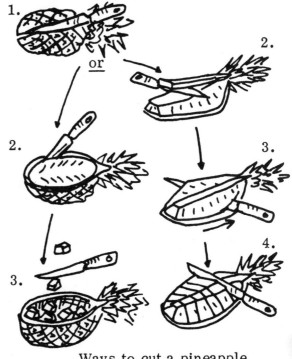

Ways to cut a pineapple

SALAD OF THE GODS

3 C pineapple
3 oranges
3 bananas
3 avocados

3 T honey
3 T shredded coconut
3 T pecans, chopped

Dice fruit and mix in the honey. Serve in dessert bowls, and sprinkle each with coconut and pecans. For 4 - 6.

MELON SALADS

MELON SALADS

1/4 honeydew melon
1/2 cantaloupe
1/2 sugar melon

1/2 casaba melon
1/2 persian melon

Cut the rinds off the melons, deseed, and slice. Arrange the slices on salad plates, and serve chilled. For 4 - 6. Use any types of ripe melons.

103

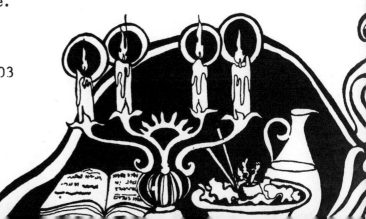

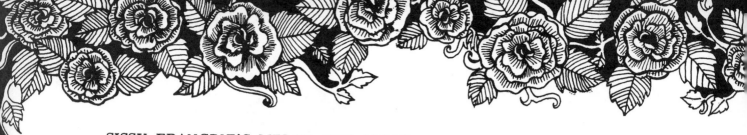

SISSY FRANCINE'S MELON FOR MANY

1 watermelon, very ripe   3-4 medium cantaloupes   2 honeydew melons

The basket

On the uncut watermelon carefully outline with a magic marker your desired fruit basket shape.   The directions below are for a scalloped-edged fruit basket.

1.   On your melon, draw the dotted lines shown.

2.   Using a long, sharp knife, cut deeply into the melon, along the lines.

3.   After completing the cutting, deftly, with a medium firm touch, whack the center of each top piece.

4.   Carefully insert your fingers into the cutting lines, and lift off each top piece.

5.   Now, carefully cut out the fruit inside the basket handle, leaving all of the light pink and white fruit attached to the handle.

6.   Next, with a circular piece of cardboard, outline scallops around the edge of the melon. Delicately cut out the scallops.

7.   Now, make melon balls with all of the fruit inside the melon. Leave about 2" of fruit inside the shell, so that it will hold its shape.

8.   Put all the melon balls into another bowl, and pour out the alkalizing watermelon juice. If it stays in the melon, the melon balls will lose their crispness.

9.   Make melon balls out of the other melons.

10.   Place the mixed melon balls into the basket. Decorate the scallops with flowers, making holes for the stems with toothpicks. Chill the basket before serving.

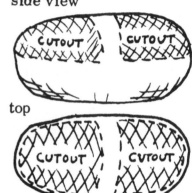

top

Step 6.

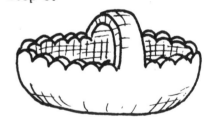

Step 10.

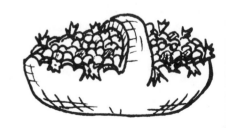

NECTARS

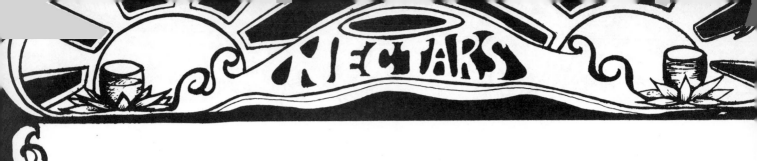

METHODS OF JUICING

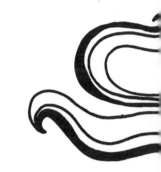

A manual grass juicer extracts juice from greens slowly, without producing heat. Without heat, nutrients are left intact, and are extracted in a form your body can quickly and easily assimilate. If there is no manual juicer available, you can run the delicate greens, or the ripe fruits and the hardier vegetables through an electric juicer. Some oxidation will occur, and some nutrients will be lost, but certainly not all.

If there is no juicer available, you can extract juice from greens, vegetables and fruits by putting them all in a blender. After reducing all to a pulp, put the pulp in a sieve, and work the juice away from the pulp with your hands. Or, instead of using a sieve, put the pulp in a large piece of cheesecloth, or a cheesecloth bag, and work the juice out of the pulp.

You can also extract juice from greens manually by grinding them between a mortar and pestle, and then putting the pulp in a piece of cheesecloth.

In summary:
1. Manual grass juicer -- excellent for juicing everything except hard root vegetables. Does not oxidize nutrients.
2. Electric juicer -- good for all juicing. Quick, efficient, easy. Does oxidize nutrients away somewhat.
3. Blender -- first blend the vegetables or fruits, then push the juice out of the pulp through a sieve, or through a cheesecloth. Some oxidation will occur in the blender, some nutrients will be lost.
4. Mortar and pestle -- more work, less juice extraction, but no oxidation will take place.
5. Chewing -- original juice extraction method. Most reliable. Just spit out the pulp.

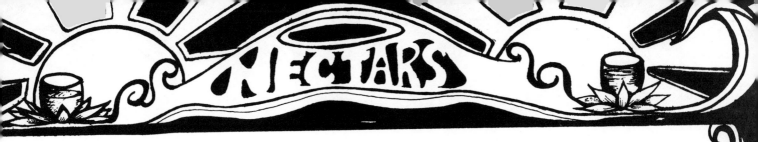

NECTARS

GREEN DRINKS

GREEN DRINK #1

2 C buckwheat lettuce
1 C sunflower greens
2 C sprouts

Juice it all, and drink the liquid chlorophyll. Makes about 8 oz.
Use any kind of greens you have on hand, and any sprouts. Spice
your green drink up with a clove of garlic, or a teaspoon of cayenne
pepper. Add in any vegetables you have on hand.

SPIRITUAL DRINK

1 C sunflower greens   4 T sauerkraut (optional)
1 C buckwheat greens   1 stalk celery
1 C alfalfa sprouts   1 sprig parsley
2 T fenugreek sprouts   1/2 C spinach leaves
1 clove garlic   1 C favorite weeds (optional)

Run all through a manual grass juicer, or see previous page on
methods of juicing. To get all the juice out, run it through more than
once. It has a salty, very agreeable taste. To sweeten the drink,
add an equal amount of carrot juice. Without the carrot juice, the
recipe makes about 8 oz.

GREEN DRINK #2

1 small bunch wheatgrass   2 C indoor salad greens
2 C mixed sprouts - alfalfa, mung.   1/2 C fenugreek sprouts

Juice all in a grass juicer, or blend the greens, place in a cheesecloth bag and squeeze the juice out from the pulp. Makes about 8 oz.

To make a zesty green drink, add in 2-4 cloves garlic, and 1 - 2
teaspoons of cayenne pepper.

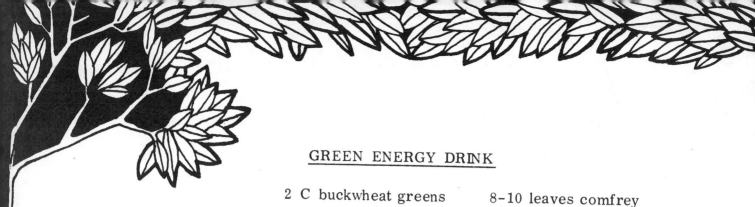

GREEN ENERGY DRINK

2 C buckwheat greens   8-10 leaves comfrey
1 small zucchini   1 C favorite weeds

Juice all. Makes about 8 oz. Use any extra greens you have on hand as well. Add in a pinch of kelp too. If your green drink needs sweetening, add in an appropriate amount of carrot juice.

VEGETABLE JUICES

These juices are most easily made in an electric juicer. Use fresh, ripe vegetables.

VEGETABLE COCKTAIL

4 ounces carrot juice
2 ounces celery juice
1 ounce tomato juice
1 ounce parsley juice

For one 8-ounce
glass.

REAL V-8 JUICE

8 ounces tomato juice
2 ounces carrot juice
1 ounce of each of these juices:
celery juice, beet juice
lettuce juice, parsley juice
watercress juice
spinach juice

CARROT SHAKE

1 C carrot juice
1 T sunflower seeds
1 T dulse
1 t honey

Blend all till smooth. 8 oz.

POTATO LIFT

1 organic potato
1 t vegetable seasoning

Scrub the potato, and remove any buds. Extract the juice, and season with the powder. Drink immediately. 4-8 oz.

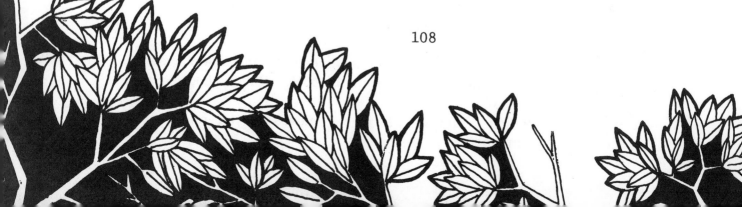

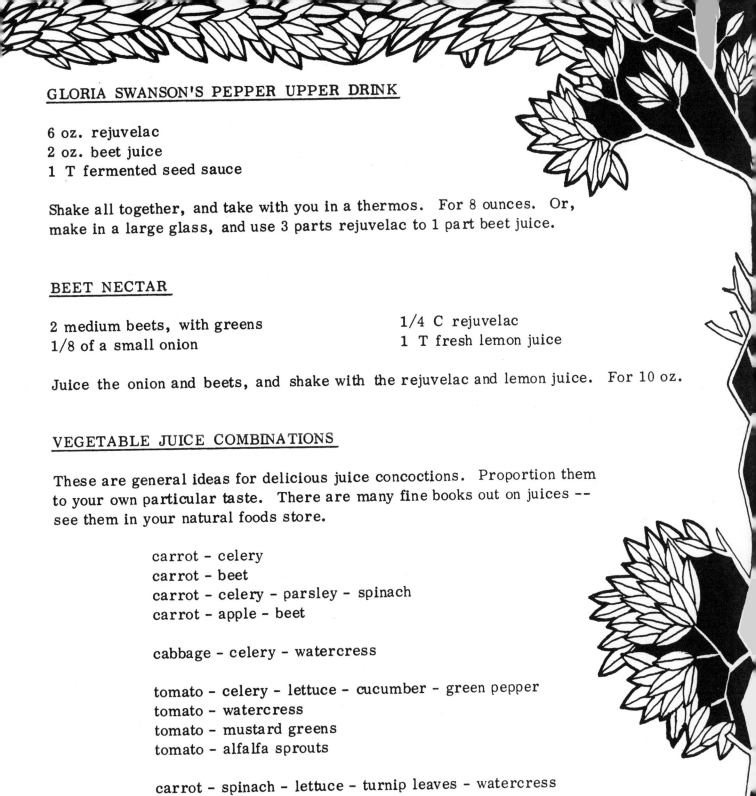

GLORIA SWANSON'S PEPPER UPPER DRINK

6 oz. rejuvelac
2 oz. beet juice
1 T fermented seed sauce

Shake all together, and take with you in a thermos. For 8 ounces. Or, make in a large glass, and use 3 parts rejuvelac to 1 part beet juice.

BEET NECTAR

2 medium beets, with greens   1/4 C rejuvelac
1/8 of a small onion   1 T fresh lemon juice

Juice the onion and beets, and shake with the rejuvelac and lemon juice. For 10 oz.

VEGETABLE JUICE COMBINATIONS

These are general ideas for delicious juice concoctions. Proportion them to your own particular taste. There are many fine books out on juices -- see them in your natural foods store.

> carrot - celery
> carrot - beet
> carrot - celery - parsley - spinach
> carrot - apple - beet
>
> cabbage - celery - watercress
>
> tomato - celery - lettuce - cucumber - green pepper
> tomato - watercress
> tomato - mustard greens
> tomato - alfalfa sprouts
>
> carrot - spinach - lettuce - turnip leaves - watercress
> carrot - turnip leaves - dandelion leaves
> carrot - cucumber
> carrot - beet - spinach

109

NUT AND SEED MILKS

NUT AND SEED MILK

    1/3 C any nut or seed: almond, sesame, brazil nut
    1 C spring water
    2 t raw honey
    1-2 drops pure vanilla extract

Grind the seeds to a meal in a nut grinder or grain mill. Blend all ingredients to a milk consistency. Makes about 1 1/2 cups.

Nut and seed milks are best used immediately, but will store, refrigerated, for 1 or 2 days.

If a blender is unavailable, shake the ground seed meal and water in a tightly capped jar.

Instead of grinding the seed first, you can add the soaked seeds to the blender. Put in the water first, then drop the seeds in bit by bit. Both methods work out well, but you will save wear and tear on the blender by grinding the seed first. For a thinner milk, pour the mixture through a sieve before drinking. Use any kind of nut or seed to make this milk, in any kind of combination.

SESAME MILK

1/2 C sesame seed   1 C water or rejuvelac
1/8 t kelp

Put the liquid in the blender, and slowly add in the seed. Blend for about 1 minute, adding in the kelp. Pour the mixture through a strainer to remove any pulp. Season to taste with additional kelp, if desired. Makes 8 ounces.

For a blander taste, try a 50-50 mixture of sesame and sunflower. You can soak the seeds overnight to reduce strain on your blender.

Try this with different seeds and nuts.

110

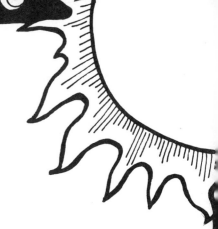

CASHEW MILK #1

1/2 C cashew nuts, soaked 8 hours
2 dates, pitted
1 C spring water

Blend and enjoy. For 8 oz. Use this as you would any other milk.

CASHEW MILK #2

1/3 C cashews
1 C pure water
1/4 C chopped dates

1/4 t dulse
1-2 drops pure vanilla extract

Grind the cashews in a nut or grain mill. Blend the meal with the other ingredients until smooth. If a blender is unavailable, shake well in a tightly capped jar, or use an egg beater. Makes about 12 oz.

WALNUT MILK

1 C spring water
2 T seed yoghurt

2 T walnut meats
2 T dates, pitted (optional)

Blend all together. Pour through a strainer before serving. If you like a thicker milk, use a bit less water. Make an almond, pecan or brazil nut milk in the same way. For 8 oz.

SOYA MILK

1 C pure water
4 T soya powder

1 T tahini
1/4 C chopped dates

Blend all. Will store in refrigerator up to 2 days. Be sure to shake well before serving. For 8 oz.

Use 4 pitted dates as a replacement for the honey,
    and/or 1 T raisins.

111

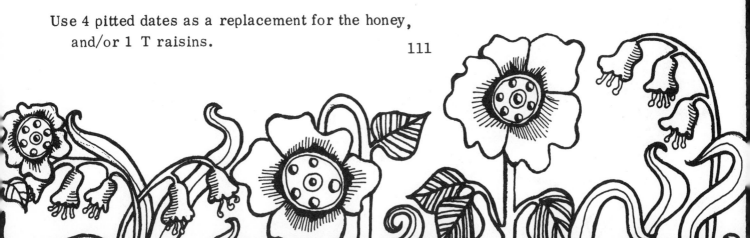

SOYBEAN MILK

1/2 pound soybeans   1 qt. spring water
2-3 T honey <u>or</u> grated coconut   1 t kelp or 1 t tamari

1. Soak the beans 48 hours. Change the water every 12 hours.
2. Grind the beans to a very fine meal, and put the meal into a cheesecloth bag.
3. Place the bag in a large bowl containing 1 quart lukewarm spring water.
4. Work the ground beans thoroughly with your hands for about 10 minutes, as if you were kneading bread. Then wring the bag of pulp until it is dry.
5. Season the milk left in the bowl to taste with the kelp/tamari, honey or coconut.
6. Makes approximately 1 quart.

WHEAT MILK

1/2 C 2-day wheat sprouts   1 T unrefined maple syrup
1 C spring water   3 dates or 3 figs (optional)

Put the water in the blender, and gradually blend in the wheat sprouts while the motor is on. Blend in the sweeteners to taste. **Strain** through a sieve. For 8 oz.

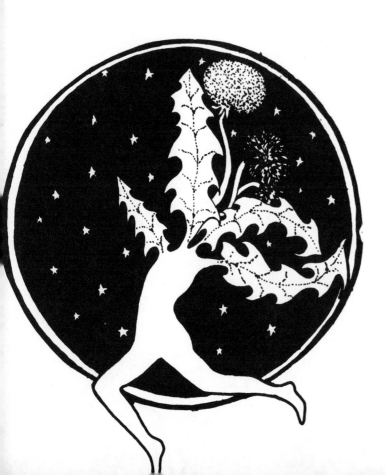

MALTED WHEAT MILK

1 1/2 C 2-day wheat sprouts
1 C spring water
3 dates, pitted
1 ripe banana, sliced
2 T carob powder

Blend the water with the sprouts, as above. Pour through a sieve, and return the liquid to the blender. Now add in the pitted dates, the sliced banana, and the carob powder. Makes about 12 oz.

"BUTTER" MILK

1 C rejuvelac
2 1/2 T fermented seed sauce
1 T raw honey (optional)

Blend all. Makes 8 oz.

112

COCONUT MILK

1 coconut
2-4 T coconut oil

spring water as needed

Open the coconut, pour out the "water" and save. Chip the meat away from the shell and skin. Pour the "water" into the blender, and gradually add in the bits of coconut meat. Keep on adding them in until you have a milk-like consistency. Make as much as you need, adding more spring water and oil to keep the texture milk-like.

You can make a rich, delicious fruit salad sauce by blending in more coconut meats and less spring water. Use it as a base for other fruit sauces; add it into the fruit smoothies following. With less liquid, it makes a great topping, in place of cream.

For a less pulpy texture, pour the liquid through a sieve to strain out pulp, or squeeze through a cloth.

COCONUT CAROB MILK SHAKE

1 C coconut milk (above)
1 T carob powder

1 t honey, or 2 pitted dates
1/8 t pure vanilla extract

Blend all. Makes 8 oz. If you have no fresh coconut milk, substitute 1/3 cup chopped nuts and one cup spring water. Place all in blender, and process until smooth.

SMOOTHIES

"Smoothies" are thick, creamy fruit drinks--made by simply blending up different chopped fruits.

Use rejuvelac or spring water as a thinner. The soak water from dried fruit is also an excellent thinner.

For sweeteners, if your drink needs one, try unrefined honey or maple syrup. Prunes, pitted dates, raisins or dried figs also add sweetness. Experiment! Just blend, and taste!

See the food combining chart at the end of the book for fruit ideas, and to see which fruits combine most harmoniously.

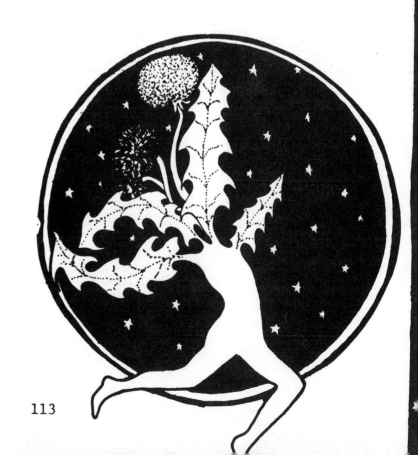

113

DATE/COCONUT SMOOTHIE

    2-4 dates, pitted
    4-6 T shredded coconut (can be dried)
  1 C coconut milk

Put the dates and coconut in the blender, cover with the coconut milk. Blend until smooth. Makes 8 oz.

If you have no fresh coconut milk, double the amount of dried, unsweetened coconut and use 1 cup of spring water.

STRAWBERRY SMOOTHIE

1 C fresh strawberries   1 C coconut milk (or nut milk)
1 T raw honey   1 frozen banana (freeze 12-24 hours)

Peel and slice the banana before freezing. Blend all ingredients until smooth. For approximately 16 oz. Try any other berry.

STRAWBERRY FRAPPE

    1 C cashew milk
     1/2 C strawberries
      1/2 C papaya chunks
     1/2 t raw honey

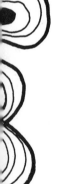

Blend all ingredients. Serve in a tall frosted glass. Makes 1 large frappe.

BERRY GOOD FRAPPE

2 C nut and seed milk (1/2 C seed meal,   1 papaya, diced
1 C fresh berries   2 C water)   8 dates, pitted

Blend all. For 2 tall glasses. Add in more nut and seed milk for a thinner frappe.

For a thicker frappe, blend in a banana. Different nut milks will provide a slight variation in flavor as well.

    Add a sprig of mint, too.

Berries
to try here:
  strawberries
  gooseberries
  blackberries
  raspberries
  blueberries
  huckle-
  berries

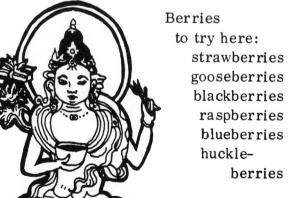

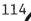
114

BANANA-MINT DRINK

2 super ripe bananas
1 C rejuvelac
2-3 fresh mint leaves

Blend bananas and rejuvelac for about 15 seconds, blend in mint. Makes about 16 oz.

MIXED FRUITS DRINK

1/2 avocado
1/2 lemon, juiced

1 1/2 C fresh pineapple, crushed
1/2 C apple juice (or apple cider)

Blend all together for a thick, creamy fruit drink. Makes about 16 oz. Add more apple juice to thin this drink.

BLUEBERRY-BANANA DRINK

1 banana
1 C blueberries

1 slice of papaya (optional)

Blend all, adding water if needed. For 1 large glass.
To make 1 1/2 quarts, use 1 box blueberries, and 6 ripe bananas.

BANANA-PEACH DRINK

1 large banana
2 small peaches

Blend both together. For 8 oz. For 1 1/2 quarts, use 5 large peaches, 6 bananas.

APPLE-GINGER NECTAR

2-3 apples
1 C water
1" piece of
  ginger root

Blend all.
For 12 oz.

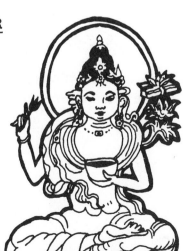

BANANA-APRICOT NECTAR

4-6 dried apricots, soaked and chopped
 1 large banana

Blend! For approximately 8 ounces.

Blend in 1 grated or chopped
 apple for a banapplicot
  nectar. Good!

115

FRUIT JUICES

These fruit juices call for a juice extractor, rather than the blender. They will be less thick than the smoothies. Try your own variations and combinations. The food combining chart will give you some ideas, perhaps, on different fruits to combine.

PINEAPPLE STRAWBERRY JUICE

2 C pineapple chunks (fresh)   8-10 fresh strawberries

Juice all -- makes about 8 ounces. For a smoothie, blend instead of juicing.

APPLE STRAWBERRY JUICE

3 medium apples   8-10 fresh strawberries

For approximately 8 ounces. Hard, firm apples make the best juice. Try various kinds of berries.

APPLE PEACH JUICE

2 large apples   2 ripe peaches

Slice the fruit, and juice. Incredibly delicious! For approximately 8 ounces.

CRANAPPLE JUICE

3 medium apples   1/2 C fresh cranberries

Juice. Makes about 8 ounces.
Apple juice combines well with just about
every other fruit juice.
Try them all!

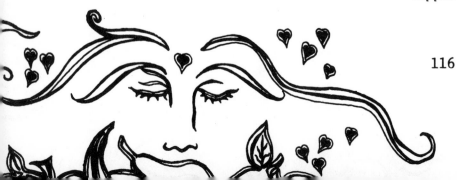

FRESH FRUIT JUICE COMBINATIONS

Each of these makes 12 ounces - enough to fill a tall glass. What a way to say "Good Morning"! Use freshly squeezed citrus juices.

8 oz. pineapple juice	9 oz. orange juice
3 oz. grape juice	2 oz. strawberry juice
1 oz. lime juice	1 oz. lime juice
5 oz. pineapple juice	4 oz. cherry juice
4 oz. orange juice	4 oz. peach juice
3 oz. lemon juice	4 oz. pear juice

ENERGIZER

1/2 C freshly squeezed orange juice	1/4 C water
1/2 C grape juice	1-2 T lemon juice

Put all these juices together in a tightly capped jar, and shake them together. This is a good "pick-me-up" and energy booster. Take it with you in a thermos, or keep on hand in the refrigerator. This makes enough to fill a large glass.

MELON-SEED DRINK

4 oz. pineapple or apple juice
3-4 C melon seeds: watermelon, cantaloupe, honeydew, plus any pulp, rinds, etc.

Juice seeds, rinds and pulp. Add fresh pineapple or apple juice. The seeds and pineapple or apple juice will make about 10 ounces.

If you use a blender, blend the seeds with the pineapple juice until they release their seed milk. Then strain out the hulls.

Add in 1 cup of pomegranate seeds for a pink color. The more pulp you add in, the sweeter the drink will be.

117

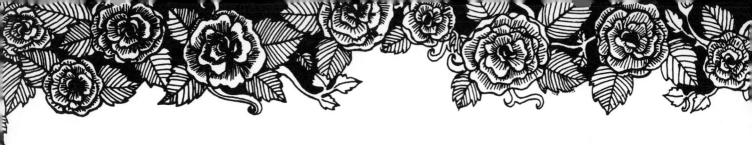

FRUIT SPECIALITIES

HERBAL APRICOT

4-5 fresh apricots, juiced   3 T freshly squeezed lemon juice
1/8 t dried tarragon

Mix the 2 fruit juices together, and stir in the tarragon. For 1 tall glass.

PINA COLADA

2 C fresh pineapple chunks   1 C fresh coconut chunks

Put all through a juicer -- for 1 tall glass.

BANANA NUT MILK

1 banana   1/4 C walnuts, pecans or cashews
1/4 C spring water   1 sprig mint

Put the water in the blender, and slowly blend in the nuts. Then, blend in the
banana. For 12 ounces, approximately.

Breakfast Ideas

BREAKFAST WATERMELON

1 big bowl of watermelon chunks - cut thickly

For 1.

Nine months out of 12, when watermelons are in season, this alkalizing, cleansing and refreshing breakfast is served at Hippocrates. It's delicious!

Juice some of the pink flesh of the melon along with the rind and drink 10-15 minutes before enjoying the rest of the watermelon.

BREAKFAST CITRUS SALAD

2 oranges   1 large grapefruit

Peel and section these fruits into wedges. Do the sectioning over the serving bowl, so that all of the fresh juice is saved, and served. For 2.

APPLE TREAT BREAKFAST

2 large apples, shredded   1/2 C sesame seed meal
1/2 C raisins, soaked   1/2 C prune juice

Blend raisins, seed and prune juice. Pour over shredded apples and serve. For 2.

PRUNE DATE BANANA BREAKFAST

4 pitted dates (or figs), soaked   2 bananas
4 large prunes, pitted, soaked

Blend soaked dates and figs in as much soak water as is needed to get a smooth sauce consistency. Serve over the sliced bananas. For 2.

AVOCADO DELIGHT

2 medium apples, chopped
1 avocado, sliced

Blend the fruit pieces together into a smooth, sauce-like consistency. For 2. Add a dash of cinnamon for more flavor.

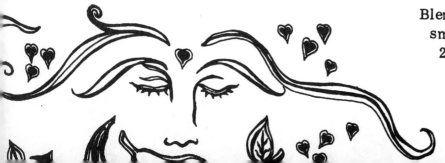

TROPICAL BREAKFAST TREAT

1/2 C raisins, soaked   1/2 C dates, soaked
1/2 C fresh coconut pieces   1 C spring water

Chop up the soaked fruit. Put the water in the blender, and slowly add in the fruit and coconut. For 2. Make this a breakfast for 4 by serving it over chopped apples.

BREAKFAST GRANOLA

1/2 C coarsely ground sesame seeds   1/2 C sprouted triticale
1/2 C coarsely ground sunflower seeds 4-8 T rejuvelac or apple juice
1 1/2 C (in any combination): raisins, dates, black mission figs, currants, banana

Mix all! Moisten with rejuvelac or apple juice. Eat as is, or blend into different variations. For 2 - 4.

SUN RISE

1/2 C sunflower seeds   1/2 C dates   1/2 C spring water

Soak the sunflower seed and dates overnight in the water. In the morning, blend all. Enjoy as is. For 2. This can also be served over chopped fruit.

WHEAT CEREAL

1 C sprouted wheat   4-5 dates, pitted   1/2 C spring water

Blend wheat and water until thick. Add dates, continue to blend until creamy. For 1.

WHEAT WITH RAISINS

1/2 C wheatberries
1/2 C unsulfured raisins

Soak the wheatberries 15 hours or more. Drain. Mix with the raisins. Chew it well. If you're in a hurry, put it in a plastic bag, enjoy it on the way to work.

121

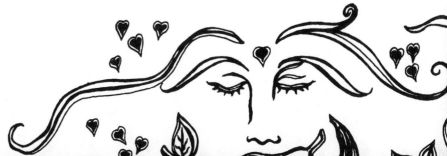

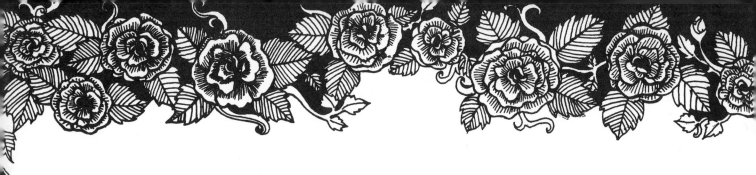

WHERE
THERE IS
FAITH
THERE IS LOVE
WHERE THERE IS LOVE
THERE IS PEACE
WHERE THERE IS PEACE
THERE IS
GOD
WHERE
THERE IS
GOD
THERE IS
NO NEED

Salad Sauces and Dressings

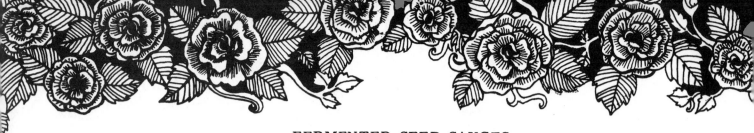

FERMENTED SEED SAUCES

See page 6 for a formal introduction to the fermented seed sauce family.

ALMOND SEED SAUCE

1 C almonds, ground to meal   2 C rejuvelac

Mix the seed meal into the rejuvelac. Put it in a covered bowl, and allow it to ferment 4-5 hours. This makes a delicious, sweetly fermented sauce. For 2 cups.

CASHEW-SUNFLOWER SEED SAUCE

1/2 C cashew meal   1/2 C sunflower seed meal   2 C rejuvelac

Mix the meal into the rejuvelac, and ferment 4-8 hours in a covered container. Replace the cashew with sesame seed meal for a different effect. Makes 2 cups.

ALMOND-SUNFLOWER SEED SAUCE

1/2 C almond meal   1/2 C sunflower seed meal   2 C rejuvelac

Ferment 4-8 hours. For 2 cups.

As you can see, it is possible to substitute any seed or any nut in any of the recipes above. Just grind the seed or nuts into a meal, and mix with the rejuvelac.

SEED & NUT SAUCES

These sauces differ mainly in that they are unfermented. They are quick and easy to prepare, and, depending on what spices you add, combine with fruit or vegetables.

SESAME SEED SAUCE

1/2 C sesame seed, ground   1 t cayenne pepper (optional)
1/2-1 C rejuvelac   1 t tamari

Blend all to a sauce consistency. Start with 1/2 cup rejuvelac; add more as needed.

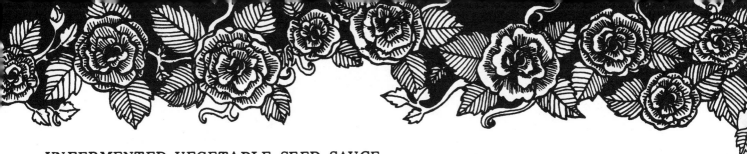

UNFERMENTED VEGETABLE SEED SAUCE

1 C sunflower seeds, soaked 24 hours   1/2 medium carrot, shredded
1/2-1 C rejuvelac   1 1/2 t kelp
1/2 beet, shredded

Blend all the ingredients to a sauce consistency, adding in rejuvelac as needed. For 2 1/2 cups, approximately.

Use any kind of soaked seed -- sesame, almond, brazil nut. Add in any kind of vegetable you may have: squash, celery, pepper.

ALMOND CREAM DRESSING

1/2 C almonds   3 T coconut oil
1 C nut milk

Make the nut milk, if you do not have some on hand, by blending 1/3 C of the nuts with 2/3-1 C water or rejuvelac. Strain out any nut pulp.

Then, blend the above ingredients together. For approximately 1 1/4 C.

SUNFLOWER SEED CREAM

1 C sunflower seeds, soaked 8-24 hours   1/8 t tamari
1/2 lemon, juiced   1/8 t kelp
1/8 t basil, sage or savory   1/4-1/2 C rejuvelac

Blend the sunflower seeds with the rejuvelac to a light consistency. Blend in the remaining ingredients. Makes about 1 cup.

For a fruit sauce, blend just the seed and rejuvelac. Add in a few dates, or a few teaspoons of honey; leave out the other seasonings.

TAHINI DRESSING

1 C tahini   1/2 C lemon juice   1 T honey (optional)

Blend all ingredients until smooth and creamy. Pour over salad. For 1 cup.

NUT CREAM DRESSING #1

1 C nut meats (sunflower, almonds,
  sesame, cashew, etc.)
1/2-1 C coconut oil
1 t tamari
3/4 C water or rejuvelac

Put 1/2 C oil and tamari in blender.
Slowly, add in nuts. Pour in oil
while motor is on -- as much as is
needed to achieve a thick, buttery
texture. (You have just made a
nut butter.)

Now, blend in the water or Rejuvelac
for a less thick sauce texture.
Delicious on a fruit or vegetable
salad. For 1 1/2 to 2 cups.

NUT CREAM DRESSING #2

1 C nut meal
1/2 C coconut oil
1/2-1 C spring water
1 t tamari
1 t kelp

Blend all ingredients. Serve
on a vegetable salad. This
makes approximately 1 1/2 cups.
For a fruit salad dressing, omit
the tamari and kelp. Instead,
add a tablespoon or so of honey.
Add in more spring water for
a thinner, more creamy texture.

YELLOW SAUCE

1/2 C grated yellow squash
1 avocado
1/2 t kelp
Water or Rejuvelac to blend

Blend all ingredients together.

LEMON OIL DRESSING

3 T lemon juice
1/2 C coconut oil
1/4 t dulse or kelp
1 T honey

Blend all ingredients together.

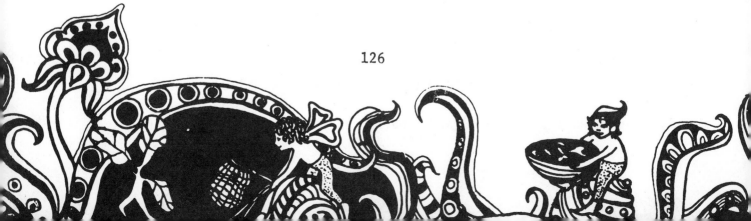

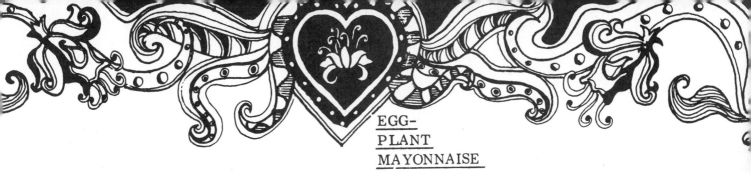

EGG- PLANT MAYONNAISE

1/2 eggplant (medium)
2 T lemon juice
2 T tahini
1/4 C cold water
3 T minced parsley

Peel and dice the eggplant.
Blend the eggplant, tahini,
and lemon juice. Use water
as needed for a smooth texture. Add in
the minced parsley for additional flavor.
This will make about 1 cup of mayonnaise.

CASHEW MAYONNAISE

1/2 C raw cashews
1 C   water
1 t kelp
1/2 t paprika
1 C coconut oil
2 lemons, juiced

Blend first 4 ingredients.
Slowly, add in the lemon
and the oil. For 4 cups.

SPECIAL AVOCADO MAYONNAISE

1-2 T coconut oil
1 C cashew nuts or pecan meats

1 T honey
1 small avocado

Grind the nuts to a meal. Put the oil in the blender, add in the avocado. Slowly, add in the nut meal, and blend until all is smooth.
Add in the honey. The avocado acts in much the same way as the oil,
giving the mayonnaise its body. Vary this dressing by adding a little
carrot or tomato juice, or a bit of onion. For approximately 1 1/2 C.

AVOCADO SAUCES

ITALIAN AVOCADO SAUCE

1 large, ripe avocado
5 T coconut oil

2 T fresh lemon juice
1/2 t fresh dill (optional)

Blend all. Makes about 1 cup. Add in more oil or lemon for a lighter dressing.

Different salad herbs -- parsley, chervil, tarragon, basil, burnet, thyme,
    fennel, mint -- will vary this dressing each time you make it.

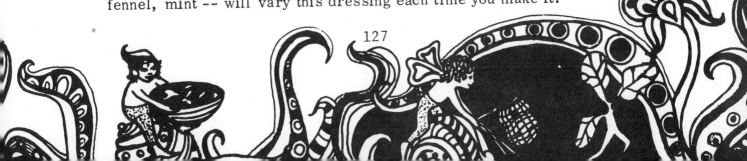

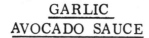

GARLIC
AVOCADO SAUCE

1 large, ripe avocado
2 cloves garlic
1-2 T coconut oil

1/4-1/2 C spring water
1/2 t kelp
1/8 t cayenne pepper

Mix all in blender, and serve chilled. Makes about 1 1/2 cups.

GUACAMOLE DRESSING #1

2 ripe avocados
1/4 C onion, diced
juice of 1 lemon

1 t cayenne pepper
1 t kelp
water as needed

Blend, using water if needed for a lighter sauce. For approximately 1 1/2 cups.

GUACAMOLE DRESSING #2

1 ripe avocado
1 diced tomato
juice of 1 lemon

1 red pepper, diced
3 T minced onion
2 T coconut oil

Slice the avocado into the blender, and process with the tomato. Add the remaining ingredients while the motor is running. For approximately 2 spicy cups of dressing.

AVOCADO-PARSLEY DRESSING

1 large, ripe avocado
1/2 medium bunch parsley

2 T tamari
1 T kelp

Cut up the parsley with scissors, add into the blender with the other ingredients. Makes about 2 cups of dressing.

COMPANY AVOCADO SAUCE

2 or 3 ripe avocados
1/2-3/4 C spring water
1 C minced parsley
2 or 3 stalks celery (including leaves)

1/2 bell pepper, chopped
1 or 2 cloves garlic, crushed
1 scallion, chopped
2 t dill

Blend the avocado with the water first to make the sauce base. Then, slowly blend in the other vegetables. Makes about 3 1/2 cups.

PURE AND SIMPLE AVOCADO SAUCE

1 ripe avocado
1/4 - 1/2 C water
1 t vegetable seasoning

Blend all until smooth. For approximately 1 cup.

TASTY DRESSINGS

PARSLEY DRESSING

1 - 3/4 C water
2 celery stalks
1/2 C coconut blended
1-3 cloves garlic
1/4 cup parsley

Blend together all
ingredients

GREEN SAUCE

1 avocado
1 T dulse
2 T chopped parsley
1 lemon juiced
Rejuvelac to blend

Blend together all
ingredients.

GINGER DRESSING

1/2 C coconut blended
3 T lime juice
Grated lime rind
1 T honey
1 T grated ginger root
1 clove garlic
1 T beet juice

Blend together all ingredients.

JOSEPH'S FAVORITE ITALIAN DRESSING

1 pint coconut oil
2 T spanish paprika
2 T crushed basil leaf
2 T Joseph's Seasoning Powder (page 37)

1/2 t crushed oregano
dash each: cayenne, kelp, thyme
1/2 t dill leaf
1/2 t minced bell pepper

Shake to mix in glass bottle.   Stand at room temperature. Use as needed along with tamari soy sauce. Excellent over sprout salads. Dressing may be thinned with water before using, if desired.

TANGY SALAD DRESSING

2/3 C coconut oil
1/3 C freshly squeezed lemon juice
1/3 C fresh pineapple juice
2 t tamari

1 t unfiltered honey
3/4 t herbal seasoning
1 fresh sweet basil leaf, chopped
1 clove garlic

Blend all ingredients. Easy to make, and tasty too! Substitute freshly squeezed orange juice for the pineapple juice if pineapples are not in season. Or, use more oil and lemon. For 1 1/3 cups.

OIL DRESSING

1 C coconut oil
1/3 C tahini (5 T)

1/2 C spring water
1 juiced lemon

2 t kelp
1 t dill

Blend well -- makes approximately 2 cups. Add in a clove of garlic for more flavor.

SUNFLOWER SEED OIL DRESSING

1/2 C coconut oil
3 T lemon juice, freshly squeezed

1 T raw apple cider vinegar
1 T unfiltered honey

Mix lemon juice, vinegar and honey. Stir in the oil. For about 3/4 cup.

130

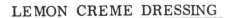

LEMON CREME DRESSING

4 T lemon juice   1 T cashew nut butter   1/2 C coconut oil

Combine lemon juice and cashew butter in blender. Add in coconut oil bit by bit. 3/4 of a cup.

JOSEPH'S SPECIAL SAUCE

1/2 C coconut oil   1 T nutritional yeast   1/2 t tamari
1/4 C soaked dulse, cut up   1-2 T kelp   1/8 t basil

Blend all well and serve over salad. Add in a pinch of oregano for variety. 3/4 cup.

SPICY FRENCH DRESSING

1/4 C apple cider vinegar   1 1/3 C coconut oil
1 medium, ripe tomato   1 t kelp
1 clove garlic   1 t cayenne
1 small onion, sliced   1 T tamari
  or 2 scallions

Blend column 1 ingredients for 1 minute to liquefy. Add in column 2 ingredients, and blend a few seconds more. This will yield 2 cups.

CHEF'S SPECIAL FRENCH DRESSING

8 T coconut oil   1 t chopped onion
4 T lemon juice, freshly squeezed   1 t honey (optional)
4 T orange juice, freshly squeezed

Shake all in a jar to blend. Makes about 1 cup of dressing.

Variation: Replace the lemon and orange juice
         with 8 T of carrot juice, or 8 T of
         tomato juice. Also try 4 T each of the
         vegetable juices.

131

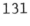

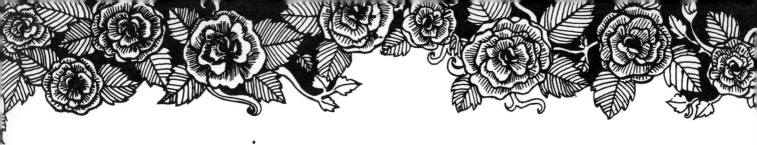

VEGETABLE SAUCES

PURE & SIMPLE VEGETABLE SAUCE

1 vegetable, chopped   coconut oil as needed   1 T kelp

Almost every vegetable can be made into a sauce either alone or in combination with others simply by placing the chopped or grated vegetables in the blender and liquefying. For example, a red sauce can be made from tomatoes, carrots, squash and beets. A green sauce can be made from parsley, celery, spinach, and avocado. Use kelp or a little oil to bind and add flavor to your sauces -- try different spices too.

You can blend in any other vegetables for additional flavors.

For a thicker sauce, add in a few tablespoons of seed meal, or a few tablespoons of oil. Avocado is an excellent binder also.

SQUASH SAUCE

1 medium squash, grated   3 fresh leaves basil
1/2 tomato   1 clove garlic
1/2 avocado   1 T coconut oil
2 scallions   1/2 t vegetable seasoning
1 stalk celery   1/4-1/2 C rejuvelac or water
1/2 bell pepper

Blend all of the above ingredients together; add liquid as needed for desired texture. Makes about 2 1/2 cups.

ZUCCHINI SAUCE

1 small zucchini squash   1/4 C coconut oil
1 stalk celery   1 T tamari
4 sprigs parsley   4-5 T water or rejuvelac

Chop and blend all ingredients, adding water as needed for sauce consistency. For 1 1/2 - 2 cups of dressing.

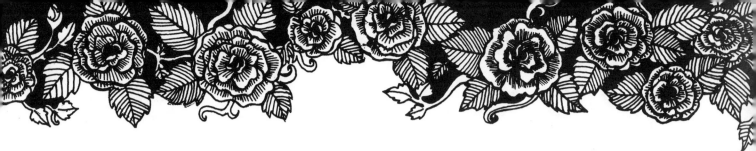

PUMPKIN OR BUTTERNUT SQUASH SAUCE

2 C grated pumpkin or squash
1/2 avocado, sliced
1/2 bell pepper, chopped
1/2-1 tomato, chopped
1 or 2 stalks celery, with leaves, sliced

2 scallions, chopped
1 T tamari
1 T kelp
1 or 2 t sweet basil
1/4-1/2 C rejuvelac or water

Put rejuvelac in blender, blend in vegetables and spices. Add 1/4 cup more liquid if you like a less thick sauce. For 2-3 cups of sauce -- enough for an 8-10 person salad. These vegetable sauces will keep, refrigerated, for several days.

GOLDEN SAUCE

2 T coconut oil
2 T water
1/2 small zucchini squash, grated
1/2 medium carrot, grated

1 stalk celery, sliced
1 t kelp
1/8 t cayenne pepper

Put oil and water in blender, blend in the other ingredients. Process until smooth. For approximately 1 1/2 cups.

CARROT-HONEY SAUCE

1 C carrot juice
2 T coconut oil

2 T minced onion
1 T honey

Blend all together, or put in a tightly capped jar and shake until mixed. For 1 cup.

CARROT-BEET SAUCE

1 C grated carrots
1/2 C beet juice, or
   1 C grated beets

1/2 C coconut oil
1 T tamari
1 T kelp

Blend all ingredients together. For 1 1/2 - 2 cups.

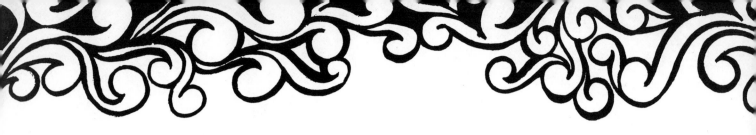

MUSHROOM SAUCE

1 C chopped mushrooms
1/4 C ground cashews
1/4 C rejuvelac or water

2 T chopped onions
1 t paprika
1-2 t tamari

Blend all together into a smooth sauce-like consistency. For 1 1/2 cups.

Variation: Add in 1 cup of alfalfa sprouts, or 1 medium tomato, or half a bunch of chopped parsley.

CORN SAUCE

2 medium cobs of corn
1 avocado, sliced

1 bunch watercress, chopped
2-3 T spring water

Cut the corn off the cob and blend with the water. Blend in the avocado and watercress, adding water if needed for a thinner sauce. Makes about 2 cups.

COUNTRY GARDEN SALAD DRESSING

4 T sunflower seed sprouts
4 T rejuvelac
1 C white cabbage
1 1/2 ripe tomatoes
1 scallion, chopped

1 T coconut oil
1/2 t dulse
1/8 t mixed herbs
pinch of cayenne

Place all ingredients in the blender in the order listed; blend until smooth. 1 cup.

CELERY SAUCE

3-4 stalks celery
1/4 C coconut oil

1 ripe tomato
2 T tamari

Blend all until smooth. For approximately 2 cups. Try adding in parsley sprigs.

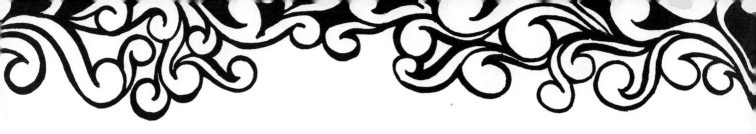

COMPANY SAUCE

1/2 C water or rejuvelac
1/2 C coconut oil
1/2 C sunflower seed meal
1/2 C beet juice (or 3/4 C grated beets)

1/4 C tamari
3 cloves garlic
1 T kelp
1 C homemade sauerkraut (optional)

Blend all the ingredients. Makes 2 cups. Delicious!

TOMATO SAUCES

ITALIAN TOMATO SAUCE

2-3 medium tomatoes, chopped
1 C almond meal
1 clove pressed garlic

2 t oregano
2 t coconut oil
2 t tamari

Blend the tomatoes, add in remaining ingredients. Pour in additional oil if needed for smoothness. Makes 1 1/2-2 cups of sauce.

TOMATO CREME DRESSING

3 ripe tomatoes, cut in pieces
2 T lemon juice

1 t cashew nut butter
1 t coconut oil

Blend all ingredients until smooth. Makes approximately 1 cup of dressing. Use any kind of nut butter for different flavors.

TOMATO-PARSLEY DRESSING

2 medium tomatoes   1/2 bunch parsley, chopped   1 t kelp

Chop the tomatoes, and blend with the parsley. Add in the kelp. For 1 1/2-2 cups.

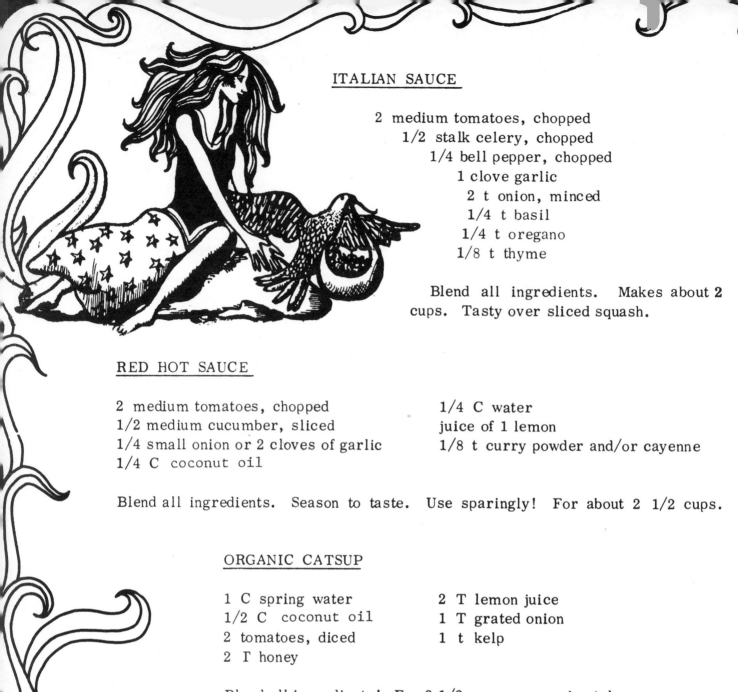

ITALIAN SAUCE

2 medium tomatoes, chopped
1/2 stalk celery, chopped
1/4 bell pepper, chopped
1 clove garlic
2 t onion, minced
1/4 t basil
1/4 t oregano
1/8 t thyme

Blend all ingredients. Makes about 2 cups. Tasty over sliced squash.

RED HOT SAUCE

2 medium tomatoes, chopped
1/2 medium cucumber, sliced
1/4 small onion or 2 cloves of garlic
1/4 C coconut oil

1/4 C water
juice of 1 lemon
1/8 t curry powder and/or cayenne

Blend all ingredients. Season to taste. Use sparingly! For about 2 1/2 cups.

ORGANIC CATSUP

1 C spring water
1/2 C coconut oil
2 tomatoes, diced
2 T honey

2 T lemon juice
1 T grated onion
1 t kelp

Blend all ingredients! For 2 1/2 cups, approximately.

TOMATO VEGETABLE SAUCE

2 medium tomatoes, chopped   1 C any sliced or diced vegetable

Blend the ingredients -- the tomatoes are a good watery base. Add seasoning.

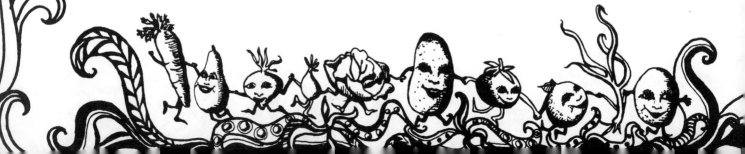

GREEN SAUCES

GREEN SAUCE

1 1/2 C chopped greens
1 C water (or less)
1/2 avocado

For the greens, use two or more
varieties that are in season. Swiss
chard and spinach, beet tops, celery,
and celery leaves produce very tasty combinations. With the water in the blender, add in
the greens a little at a time. Reduce to a fine consistency.
Add in more greens if the sauce is too thick. Add in the avocado and season to
taste with kelp or a vegetable seasoning. Serve with a vegetable salad or sprouts.
Optional -- blend in three mint leaves or the juice of half a garlic clove, one small
onion or three scallions. For 1 1/2 cups of dressing.

GREEN HERBAL SALAD DRESSING

1 1/2 C greens - any type (dandelion leaves, romaine, chicory, watercress)
1/3 C lemon juice, freshly squeezed
1/3 C coconut oil
1/2 avocado
1 clove garlic, pressed
1/2 t each: thyme, sweet basil, marjoram, tarragon

Blend all ingredients well. For approximately 1 1/2 cups.

CHLOROPHYLL SAUCE

2 C indoor greens
1 C water
1/2 avocado

4 T sunflower seed meal
1 T kelp
1 T freshly minced parsley

Pour the water into the blender, add in the remaining ingredients. For 1 3/4 cups.

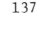

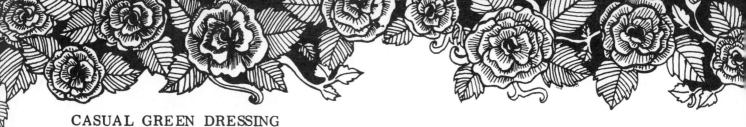

CASUAL GREEN DRESSING

1/2 C   coconut oil
3 T lemon juice
1 C greens: buckwheat lettuce, sunflower greens, parsley, comfrey, sorrel

Blend all together well. For 1 1/2 cups.

SPINACH DRESSING

1 C spinach leaves
1/2 bunch watercress
1 avocado

1/2 C spring water
1/8 t ginger
1/8 t kelp

Blend the avocado with the water; add in the remaining ingredients. For 1 3/4 cups.

COMFREY DRESSING

1 1/2 C comfrey leaves, torn
1/2 C coconut oil
1 lemon, juiced

1 T almond seed meal
1 T kelp (optional)

Blend all ingredients.   For 1 cup.

WILD EDIBLE DRESSING

1 1/2 C wild edibles: dandelion leaves, lambsquarter, purslane, chicory
1 avocado
1/2 C water
1/2 C alfalfa sprouts

Blend all together. Add seasonings as desired. For about 2 cups.

SPROUT DRESSING

2 C sprouts: alfalfa, mung, lentil
1/4 avocado
1/4 C water

4 T lemon juice
1/2 bunch watercress or parsley
1 T kelp

Put water in blender first, gradually add in remaining ingredients. For about 2 cups.

FRUIT
SAUCES

PLEASE NOTE: Calories listed in the following foods are approximated, based on information from "Composition and Facts About Foods," by Ford Heritage (Woodstown, N.J., 1968). Bear in mind that they are merely guidelines, as caloric content of foods can vary considerably. Foods grown organically, while frequently smaller than those grown in chemically treated soil, are more nutritious. Caloric variation also occurs among organically grown foods themselves and depends on richness of soil and whether or not soil is balanced (with the aid of earthworms.

QUANTITY	FOOD (UNCOOKED)*		CALORIES
	FRUITS		
1 whole	Banana		180
1 whole	Apple, Pear, Orange	(each)	100
4 oz.	Grapes		67
4 oz.	Dried Fruit		275
	VEGETABLES		
1 whole	Avocado		180
1 whole	Jerusalem Artichoke		40
1 whole	White Potato w/skin		80
1 whole	Sweet Potato w/skin		125
4 oz.	Beets		43
4 oz.	Carrots		43
4 oz.	Spinach		25
	JUICES		
16 oz.	Carrot & Beet		235
1 qt.	"Green Drink"		800
2 oz.	Wheatgrass Juice		60
	SPROUTS AND SEEDS		
4 oz.	Seed Cheese		800
6 oz.	Sprouted Wheat		435
8 oz.	Sprouts (alfalfa, mung, fenugreek, radish)		100

*Calorie counts are altered by cooking and other processing.

NUT CREAM SAUCES FOR FRUITS

ANY NUT CREAM SAUCE

1 1/2 C nut or seed meal   1/4-1/2 C coconut oil
1/2-1 C liquid

First, make your own nut butter by blending the seed meal and oil to a thick, buttery consistency. Each type of nut has a different oil content -- and will require a different amount of oil. Start off by putting 1/4 C oil in the blender (use a bit less oil for nuts that have high oil percentages -- brazil nuts, pecans, walnuts, cashews). Blend in the seed meal until you have a nut butter.

For the nut cream sauce, blend in the liquid -- rejuvelac, water, fruit juice or soak water. A dab of honey will sweeten your sauce. For about 2 cups.

Try different combinations of nuts (almond-pumpkin seed, cashew-pine nut, walnut-pecan) with coconut oil.

CASHEW CREAM SAUCE

1/2 C cashew pieces, soaked
1/2 C rejuvelac
1/2 C apple juice

Blend all. Use over a sub-acid fruit salad. For approximately 1 cup.
Try different seeds and seed meals.

WALNUT CREAM SAUCE

1/2 C walnut meats, ground
1 C rejuvelac
1 apple, chopped
1/8 t ginger

Blend the walnut meal with the rejuvelac, and blend in the apple pieces and ginger. Serve over a sub-acid/sweet fruit salad.
For about 1 1/2 cups.

Try blending in different fruits with the walnuts.

141

SWEET FRUIT SAUCES

PAPAYA DRESSING

1 sliced papaya   1/4 C spring water

Blend the papaya pieces in the water. Use over any fruit combination. 1 1/2 cups.

Variation: Add in the juice of 2 oranges instead of the water. Try this with any kind
of fruit juice -- prune juice, apple juice, pear juice, strawberry-apple juice,
apricot nectar.

PRUNE-DATE DRESSING

5 pitted dates, soaked
5 pitted prunes, soaked
1/2 C soak water (from the dates and prunes)

Blend all. Makes about 1 1/2 cups of dressing. Use over a sub-acid and/or sweet
fruit combination. Delicious over sliced bananas.

Make a banana pudding by blending the bananas into the dressing. Freeze the pudding
to make an ice cream.

APRICOT-BANANA SAUCE

5-6 dried apricots, soaked
1 banana, sliced
1/2 C soak water

Blend! Use over a sub-acid/sweet fruit combination. For about 2 cups.

For spiciness, add in a pinch of either: allspice, cinnamon, cloves or ginger.
Try this with fresh apricots as well, or use different kinds of dried fruit: dried pears,
apples, raisins.
In place of the banana, use a mango.
A few nut meats will add heaviness to this fruit sauce.
Blend in a mint leaf or two for a tangy flavor.
Make this into an ice cream by freezing, and then reblending.
Instead of a dressing, you can use this, and almost all of these sauces, as a soup.

SUB-ACID SWEET FRUIT SAUCES

CRANBERRY/BANANA DRESSING

1/3 C cranberries
2 bananas, sliced
1/4-1/2 C rejuvelac

Blend until smooth. Makes about 2 cups.

CRANAPPLE DRESSING

1/4 C cranberries
2 apples, chopped
1/4-1/2 C rejuvelac

Blend till smooth. For about 2 cups. Add more liquid if needed.
Try different kinds of liquid: soak water, spring water, fruit juices.

PRUNE-APPLE SAUCE

4 prunes, soaked
2 apples, cut up
1/4-1/2 C prune soak water

Blend all -- makes about 2 cups.
Substitute various kinds of dried fruits for the prunes.
A pinch of cinnamon or ginger will alter the taste of this sauce.
Increase the amount of water for a thinner sauce.

AVOCADO-BLUEBERRY SAUCE (*****)

1 avocado, peeled and sliced
1 C blueberries
1/2 C spring water

Blend all until smooth, creamy and velvety. Makes about 2 tasty cups of sauce.
Try a tiny pinch of ginger for spice.

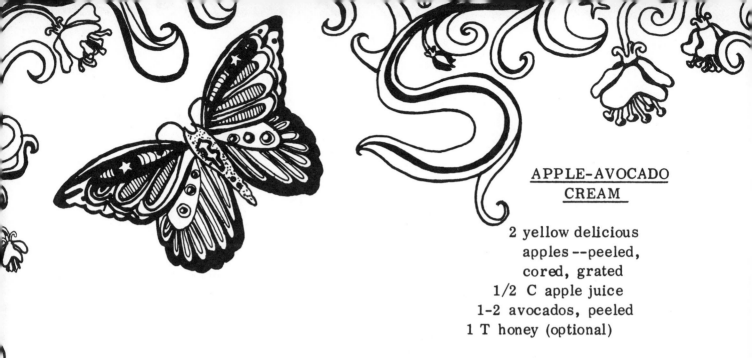

APPLE-AVOCADO CREAM

2 yellow delicious
  apples --peeled,
  cored, grated
1/2 C apple juice
1-2 avocados, peeled
1 T honey (optional)

Blend the apples with the apple juice till smooth. Then add the avocado(s). Add in the honey, if desired. Makes about 2 cups. For sub-acid fruit combinations.

CASHEW-APPLE CREAM

1 C cashews, soaked about 12 hours
2 yellow delicious apples -- peeled, cored, grated
1/2 C rejuvelac

Blend all to a creamy consistency. Makes about 2 cups.
For variety, try different kinds of apples.

CITRUS SAUCES

ORANGE SAUCE

2 oranges, freshly squeezed
  2 T coconut oil
  1 T honey

Mix the oil and honey into the orange juice. Serve over a citrus fruit salad. This sauce is delicious over sliced grapefruit.

If you desire a Thicker sauce, blend in an avocado.

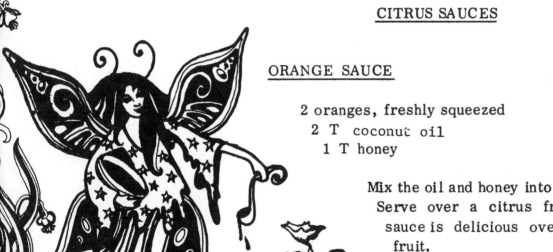

144

CREAMY CITRUS SAUCE

1/3 C sunflower seeds,
  soaked
1/2 C spring water
2 T honey
1/2 C fresh orange juice
2 t grated orange rind
2 T freshly squeezed lemon juice

Blend the sunflower seeds with the water until creamy, adding more water if needed. Add in the honey, orange peel and part of the orange juice. Gradually add in the remaining fruit juice. Blend until light. Makes about 1 1/4 cups. This sauce is good over any kind of fruit salad.

PINEAPPLE-AVOCADO SAUCE

2 C fresh pineapple chunks, crushed
3/4 C cashew nuts or pecans, soaked
1-2 T coconut oil
1 T honey (optional)
1/2 - 1 avocado

Place the first four ingredients in the blender, run about 2 minutes until the nuts are well liquefied. Add the avocado and blend for about a minute, until the dressing is emulsified. The avocado acts much the same as salad oil, giving the dressing the necessary body.

Many variations of this dressing may be made by varying the ingredients and proportions. Just the pineapple and avocado make a simple fruit dressing that is rich tasting and delicious. Use over any kind of fruit salad. The recipe above makes about 3 thick cups of sauce.

Add water or rejuvelac for a thinner sauce.
In place of the honey, add in a few T's of freshly grated coconut.

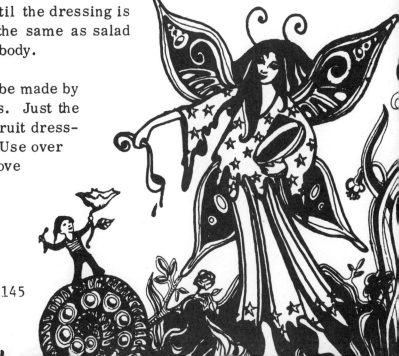

145

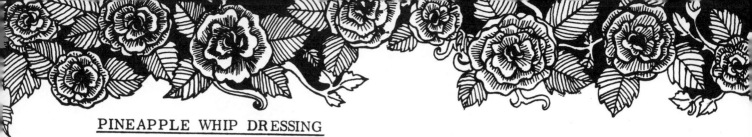

PINEAPPLE WHIP DRESSING

1/4 of a fresh pineapple
2-3 sliced bananas

Cut up the pineapple into small chunks, and liquefy the pieces in the blender. Add in the banana slices (approximately 1 banana per cup of pineapple mixture), and reblend. Makes about 3 cups of dressing.

For a less thick dressing, put the pineapple meat through a juicer. Then, blend in the banana slices.

You could serve this dressing as a soup -- topped with a few grapes.

SUGGESTIONS FOR MAKING A JELLO TREAT

The jello must be in a natural form, such as agar-agar. There are many other kinds on the market which can be purchased, and these are jellies to be used for special treats. They can be made with various kinds of fruits, especially oranges and lemon or any other kind of acid fruit. Honey can be also used. You can also make a prune jelly, which is very healthful for the children, and you can create some jelly vegetable dishes. Many other kinds of decorative dishes can be used and made into forming a salad. There are unlimited ways that jello can be used, so do experiment with it.

Celebration Food

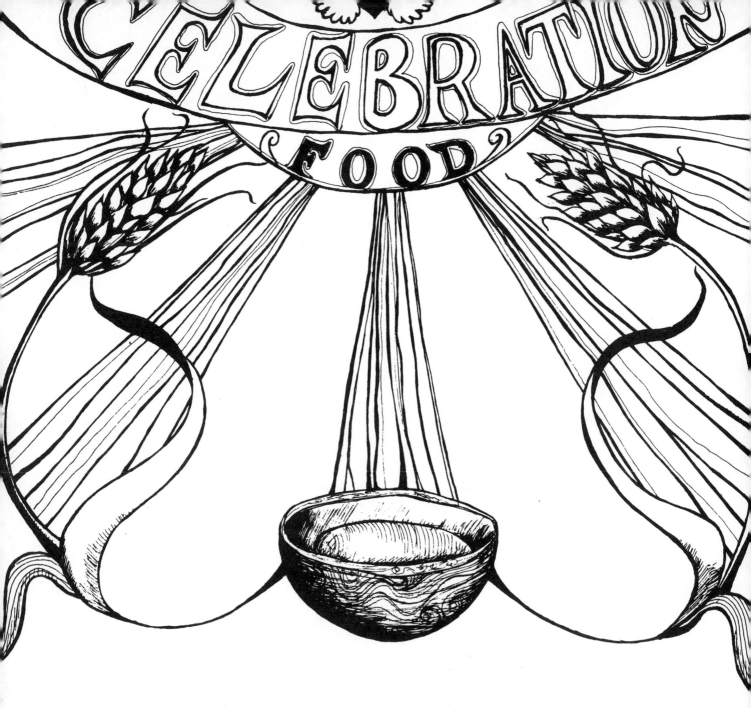

ESSENE BREAD

4 C soaked wheatberries
1/2 - 1 C finely minced vegetables (parsley, celery, onion, green pepper, carrots)
2 T seasonings (caraway seed, poppy seed, sesame seed, garlic)

Soak wheat in water at least 15 hours. Pour off water and allow wheat to drain for 15 hours. Or, better still, use the wheatberries left from making a week's supply of rejuvelac.

Put wheatberries through the Champion juicer or a hand grinder. Add vegetables -- sprinkle seasonings on top of the "bread." Form into a loaf or patties. Bake in sun or warm place (on top of a radiator) (70-90 degrees) until firm. It may be necessary to turn the loaves a few times so that the underside does not stay sticky. "Bake" about 12-24 hours. The longer the bread sets, the stronger the flavors will become.

148

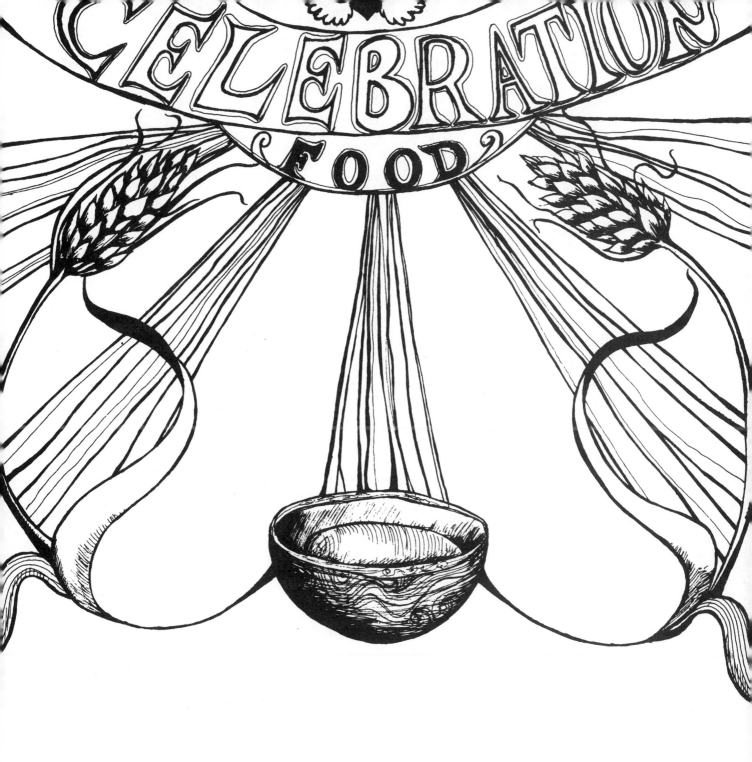

PIZZA

1 chapati (page 150)
1 C tomatoes, chopped
1/2 C peppers, chopped
1/2 C mushrooms, sliced
any other favorite uncooked
    pizza ingredient

2-3 T coconut oil
1-2 T tamari
1 T basil
1-2 t Joseph's Seasoning
1 t oregano
pinch of cayenne pepper

Sprinkle one chapati with olive oil, rub tamari over that, and sprinkle on spices and herbs. Add the raw pizza ingredients, remaining coconut oil, and enjoy! For 2 - 4.

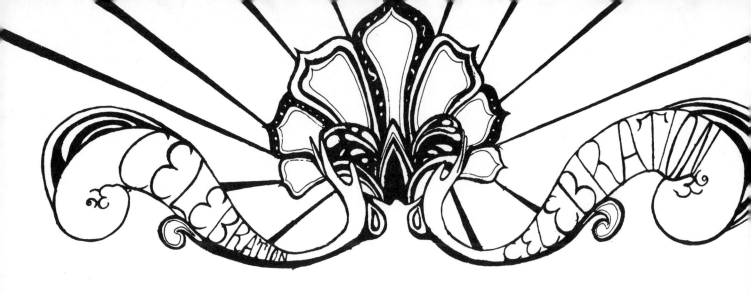

LIVING BREAD (CHAPATIS)

4 C organic wheatberries, or triticale, sprouted
8-9 T sesame seed
1-2 T coconut oil

Soak 2 cups of triticale or wheat overnight in just enough water to cover. Drain the water, refrigerate and use for drinking or dressings. Keep the grain in a loosely covered glass jar for one day, in the sun if possible. The next morning, run the grain through a food homogenizer (the Champion juicer, a Health Fountain juicer, a meat/food grinder) or pound with a wooden mortar and pestle into a smooth dough.

Oil a flat large plate with coconut oil and sprinkle thickly with sesame seed. Form round, flat chapatis with your hands, and press them out to 1/4 inch thickness. Oil your hands before working with the dough.

Set the chapatis in a sunny window, or outdoors in the full sun, or in a warm, dry place in the house (near a hot air vent, over a radiator, etc.). After 6 hours or so, loosen the chapati with a flat butcher knife, and turn it over into another plate. (Just place another plate over the chapati and turn the two plates over.) Now, allow the other side to dry or sun bake.

Allow your living bread to dry completely in the sun or indoors. Refrigerate until ready to eat (stored in a plastic bag). Chapatis may be kept indefinitely in paper or plastic bags for use on camping trips, picnics, travel, etc.

You can make a different flavored bread by using a mixture of other grains: rye, buckwheat, corn, millet, rice, etc. This recipe makes 2 or 3 chapatis.

Add additional flavor to your loaves by mixing into the dough, or sprinkling on top:

whole poppy seeds	whole or ground caraway seeds
tamari	tahini, or any nut butter
garlic	any spice
any ground seed -- brazil nuts, pumpkin seeds, sunflower seeds	

150

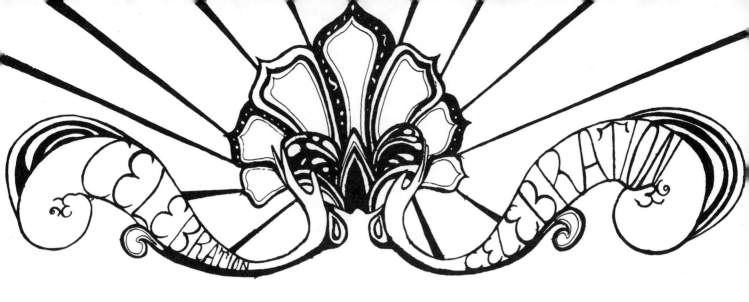

GUACAMOLES

GUACAMOLE #1

1-2 avocados
1/2 red bell pepper
1 tomato
1 clove garlic (optional)

1/2 summer squash, grated
1/2 green pepper, minced
1 tomato, chopped
2 t kelp

Blend column 1 vegetables in blender, until smooth. Pour into serving bowl, and mix column 2 vegetables into the guacamole. Serve as a dip, or as a side dish. This makes about 3 1/2 cups.

GUACAMOLE #2

1 ripe avocado
2 diced tomatoes

1 lemon, juiced
1 red pepper, diced

onion or garlic to taste
1-2 T vegetable seasoning

With a fork, blend the avocado to a creamy consistency. Combine with all other ingredients, saving some tomatoes to sprinkle on top. This can be served as a raw sandwich on a lettuce leaf, or as a stuffing for a hollowed-out tomato or pepper. Use as a dip for raw vegetables. This recipe will make about 3 cups.

Variations: Add in 1 small spanish onion, diced; freshly minced chili pepper, the juice of a clove of garlic. Combine with celery or mung sprouts for a salad.

GUACAMOLE #3

1 avocado
1 diced tomato
2 T coconut oil

1 T kelp
1 t cayenne pepper
1 t Joseph's seasoning (see page 28)

Mash the pitted avocado, and mix to a creamy consistency -- leave in a few lumps for texture. Mix in the other ingredients.

SEED CHEESES AND LOAVES

SEED LOAF

1 C ground sesame seed
1 C ground sunflower seed
1/2 C ground cashew nuts
1/3 C rejuvelac
1/2 small onion, chopped
1 stick celery, chopped

1/2 bell pepper, chopped
5-6 mushrooms, chopped
4-5 T minced parsley
1 T each: thyme, oregano, basil
         ground caraway
1-2 T kelp

Mix all ingredients together. Add more rejuvelac, if needed, to achieve a gummy consistency. Shape into a loaf, place on a plate and cover with a clean cloth. Place in a warm place (on top of a radiator, in the sun, in a food dehydrator) from 24 - 48 hours, until the flavors are well-combined (taste to tell).

To serve, shape into little balls and place on a serving platter. Or, stir in 1 or 2 blended tomatoes. Use this creamier mixture as a stuffing for celery stalks, cherry tomatoes, pepper slices.

RAW VEGETABLE NUT LOAF

1/2 C ground carrots
1/2 C finely chopped tomatoes
1/2 C finely chopped celery
1/4 C minced parsley
1/4 C minced bell pepper

2 T coconut oil
1 clove crushed garlic
3 C ground nut meal (almond, sesame,
         pignolia, sunflower) in any ratio
1/2 C rejuvelac

Mix the nut meal and vegetables -- add rejuvelac to get a doughy texture. Form into a loaf, and cover with a damp, clean cloth. Allow to set 48 hours for full permeation of flavors; good also after one day. Use the taste test! Very rich! For 1 loaf. Vary the taste of this loaf by fermenting the nut meal and rejuvelac alone, and then adding in the minced vegetables.

Make this a lighter loaf by adding in 3 or 4 homogenized carrots after fermentation. Serve inside rolled lettuce leaves, or rolled up in soaked hiziki strips.

Add 2 or 3 homogenized, or blended, beets to the loaf for a pink color and a lighter texture. You can use this as a dip for a platter of raw vegetables.

VEGETABLE/SEED CHEESE

1 C almonds, ground
1 C sunflower seed, ground
2 C rejuvelac
1 T kelp
1 T basil

4-5 T minced carrots
4-5 T minced beets
3 T minced onions
4-5 T minced celery
2 T tamari

Mix all, making sure vegetables are well chopped. Ferment 14 hours. Use this to stuff celery. Put the celery stalks in a salad, or serve as an appetizer. See page 10 for additional ideas on how to make and use seed cheese.

NUT AND SEED PATTIES

2/3 C mushrooms, chopped
1/2 C chopped onions
1/2 C ground sunflower seed
1/2 C ground almonds or pine nuts
1/3 C minced parsley

1/2 C seed cheese
6 T tahini
2 T lemon juice
1/2 - 1 C sesame seed
1 summer squash (optional)

Mix together all ingredients. Shape into patties. Coat with sesame seeds. Makes about 2 dozen small patties. Serve on top of a squash slice, or a zucchini round.

NUT SAVOURY

1 C ground nuts: almond, cashew, pignolia
4 T coconut oil
4 T finely grated carrot

2 T freshly chopped chives, scallions
1/4 t kelp
1/4 t curry powder

Stir these ingredients together; press into cakes or balls. Serve as is. Makes about 1 dozen small cakes.

COTTAGE NUT CHEESE

1 C cashew nuts
1 C spring water

Soak the cashew nuts in the water over-night. Put the soak water in the blender, and drop in the nuts bit by bit. Set in warm, dry spot for 24 hours. Use as you would use cottage cheese.

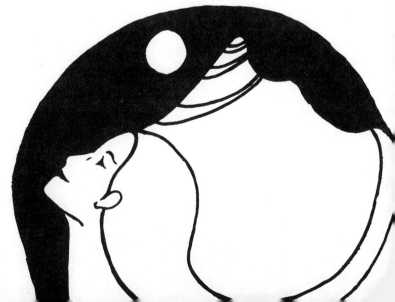

153

CHICK PEA DIPS AND SPREADS

CHICK PEA COTTAGE CHEESE

1 C 2-day chick pea sprouts
1 C spring water
1/4 C freshly squeezed lemon juice

Blend chick peas with water (use soak water for additional nutrition). Add the lemon juice. Blend until thick. Tastes much like cottage cheese and is high in protein. For approximately 1 1/2 cups. For additional flavor, blend in 2 or 3 T's of minced pepper; 1 or 2 T's of minced garlic; 1/2 t kelp; 1/8 t cayenne.

GARBANZO DIP

1/4 C coconut oil   1/2 C sesame seed
1/4 C lemon juice   1 T tamari
2 C chick pea sprouts

Place the liquids in the blender. Slowly, drop in chick pea sprouts while motor is on. Process until very smooth. Delicious! For about 2 cups of dip. Make this into a sauce by adding rejuvelac. Turn it into humus by adding 1/4-1/2 cup of tahini.

HUMUS

2 C chick pea sprouts   1/4 C coconut oil
1 C water   1/4 C freshly squeezed lemon juice
1/4 C tahini (8 T)   3-4 T tamari

Puree the sprouts, and then blend in the other ingredients.
For approximately 3 cups. Add garlic to taste.

154

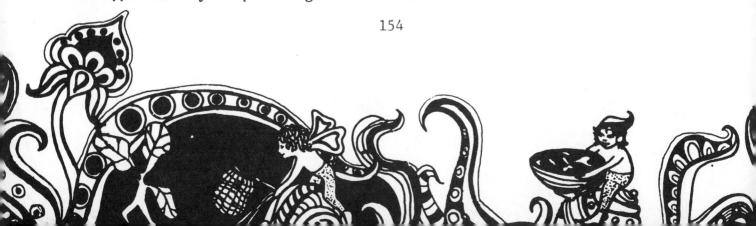

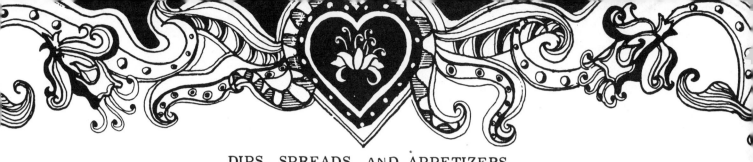

DIPS, SPREADS, AND APPETIZERS

VEGETARIAN CHILI DIP

1 medium green pepper
1 blended tomato

1/2 C almond meal
1 T cayenne pepper, or chili powder
2 C diced tomatoes

Blend all ingredients, except for diced tomatoes. Stir them in by hand. Use for a raw vegetable dip, or as a heavy salad dressing. For 2 cups.

FRESH VEGETABLE APPETIZER SAUCE

1 large tomato, blended
1 T freshly grated horseradish
1 T apple cider vinegar

2 T lemon juice
2 T finely minced celery

Blend all ingredients. Chill before serving. For about 2 cups.

FRESH VEGETABLE APPETIZER CUP

1/2 C finely diced raw carrot
1/2 C finely diced celery
1 T diced green pepper

1/2 C diced fresh tomato
1/2 C diced raw cauliflower
    (or any uncooked vegetable)
Appetizer Sauce (above)

Mix all ingredients, and serve well chilled in stemmed glasses. Serves 4.

You can try any other dip in place of the appetizer sauce above. Or, make this a platter dish by putting the sauce in a bowl, and surrounding the bowl with finger-sized pieces of the vegetables.

Sprinkle kelp over the top of each glass for more spiciness.

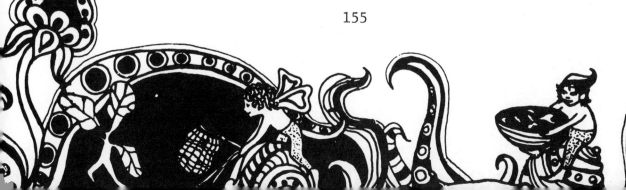
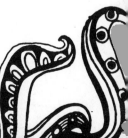

CUCUMBER-CASHEW SANDWICH

1 cucumber, finely chopped
1/2 C cashews, ground
1/2 avocado, mashed

1/2 t mixed herbs--thyme, chervil
1/2 bell pepper, finely chopped
8 stalks celery

Mix all ingredients together into a smooth spread. Fill celery sticks, or spread on cabbage or lettuce leaves. Roll the leaves, and fasten with toothpicks.

SEED DIP

1/2 C seed (sunflower, almond, sesame, pumpkin)
1-2 C warm water or rejuvelac
1 C indoor greens (or any green, torn into bite size pieces)
1 C grated squash: summer, zucchini, hubbard, crook neck
1-2 T onion, minced
1 t garlic, minced
1/2 t cayenne pepper

Soak seed overnight, and blend with 1 cup of water until smooth (process at least one minute). Or, grind the dry seed to a meal, and blend with the water until creamy. Blend in the remaining ingredients. Add more seed for a thicker consistency. For a more spicy tang, add more onion, garlic, chili or cayenne pepper. You can also transform this dip into a seed sauce by adding more rejuvelac. For about 2 cups.

THE GREEN DIP

1/4 C watercress leaves
1/2 medium cucumber
1 scallion
1/4 C wheat sprouts

2 T fermented seed cheese
1/2 clove crushed garlic
1 T tamari
1/8-1/4 C water

Finely chop watercress, cucumber, scallion and sprouts. Gently mix in the other ingredients. Chill and serve cold. For approximately 1 1/2 cups.

Vary this dip by blending it to create a smoother texture. Add in more greens also, and different kinds of greens -- comfrey, lambsquarter. Make this a spicy dip by using 1/4 cup of mustard greens.

156

MUSHROOM SPREAD

1 C coarsely chopped mushrooms
1 small onion, chopped

3-4 T seed sauce
1 t tamari

Blend one-half of the mushrooms and onions with the seed sauce and tamari. When smooth, gently stir in the remaining mushrooms and onions. Serve in a bowl, and surround with parsley sprigs for decoration. Makes 1 1/2 cups.

AVOCADO BALLS

1 ripe avocado
2 T coconut oil
2 T freshly squeezed lemon juice

1 clove garlic, minced
1/4 t cayenne pepper
1/4 t kelp

Remove the avocado pulp with a melon-ball scoop. Mix the remaining ingredients. Place the avocado balls in a bowl, and pour the marinade over them. Chill for several hours, stirring occasionally. Drain, insert a wooden toothpick in each, and serve! Makes about 10. Use the marinade as a salad dressing base.

ALFALFA SPROUT NIBBLES

1/2 C alfalfa sprouts
1/4 C seed meal
1/4 C rejuvelac or spring water

3-4 T chopped almonds
1 t tamari
pinch of curry powder

Coarsely chop the alfalfa sprouts. Blend the seed meal with the rejuvelac. Gently mix the alfalfa sprouts and chopped almonds into this seed cheese, and add in the spices. Roll into little balls, and chill before serving. Makes about 15 small nibbles.

PEPPER WHEAT

1 C sprouted wheat
1/2 C water or rejuvelac
1 red sweet pepper, chopped
1 T Joseph's seasoning powder
1 scallion

Blend the wheat with the water. Add in the
remaining ingredients, and reblend. For
roughly 1 1/2 cups.

157

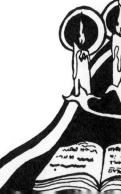
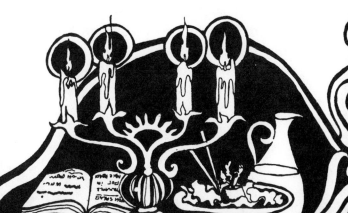

STUFFED VEGETABLES

MUSHROOM LOAF STUFFING FOR VEGETABLES

1 C sunflower seeds, ground
1/2 C almond seeds, ground
1/2 C pumpkin or sesame seeds, ground
1/3 C water or rejuvelac
3/4 C mushrooms, minced

2 T fresh parsley, minced
2 T kelp
8 celery stalks
10-12 cherry tomatoes, hollowed out
1 green pepper, sliced

Mix all but last three ingredients. Form into a loaf, and ferment 24-48 hours. Now, stuff the celery stalks, tomatoes, and pepper slices with the seed loaf. Arrange on a platter for an appetizer, or place the stuffed vegetables in a complete meal salad.

After fermentation, if you desire a lighter taste and texture, knead in a blended squash, or tomato. Or, stir in more liquid.

NUTTY CELERY STICKS

1/4 C nut butter (8 T)   2 large celery stalks

Slice the celery stalks into 3 or 4 inch pieces; put the nut butter in the middle. Good!

STUFFED CHERRY TOMATOES

10-12 cherry tomatoes
2 T   coconut oil
1/2 C lentil sprouts
1/2 C almonds, chopped (or cashews)
1 t kelp
1 t basil
2 t freshly minced parsley

Hollow out the tomatoes, and save the pulp. Blend the pulp to a liquid, and mix all the other ingredients into the blended tomato. Use this as the stuffing for the tomatoes. Add more lentils if more bulk is needed. Top with additional parsley.

158

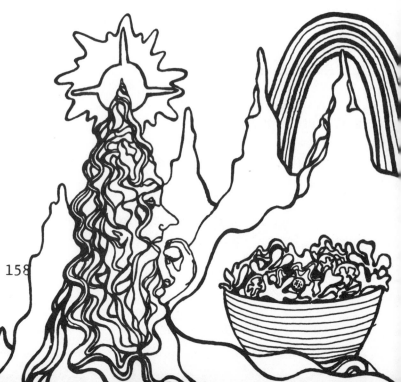

TOMATO ROLLS

1 tomato, cut into 8 wedges
4 large lettuce leaves, torn in 2

1/2 C alfalfa sprouts
1/4 C fermented seed sauce

Mix the seed sauce with the sprouts. Place 1 tomato wedge and 1/8 of the seed-sprout mixture on a lettuce leaf. Wrap the lettuce tightly around the tomato and sprouts. Fasten with a toothpick. For 8 rolls.

Try different vegetables as a stuffing--cucumber slices, potato bits, cauliflowerettes.

TABOULE STUFFED TOMATO CUPS

1 C taboule (see page 33)

10-15 cherry tomatoes

Hollow out the tomatoes, and mix the pulp into the taboule, if you like. Stuff them! Put each cherry tomato inside a tiny bibb lettuce leaf for a decorative effect.

STUFFED MUSHROOMS #1

12 large mushrooms
6 T ground sesame seed
4 T tahini

1/2 clove garlic, pressed or crushed
2 T parsley, minced
2 T freshly squeezed lemon juice

Hollow out the mushrooms. Put chopped mushroom stems and all other ingredients in a bowl. Mix to a thick, paste-like consistency, and stuff the mushroom caps with the mixture.

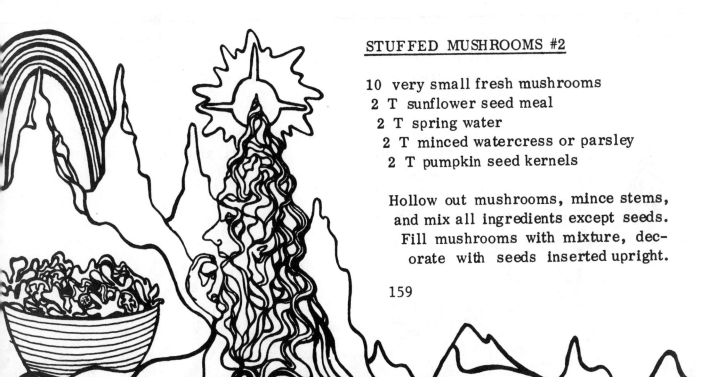

STUFFED MUSHROOMS #2

10 very small fresh mushrooms
2 T sunflower seed meal
2 T spring water
2 T minced watercress or parsley
2 T pumpkin seed kernels

Hollow out mushrooms, mince stems, and mix all ingredients except seeds. Fill mushrooms with mixture, decorate with seeds inserted upright.

159

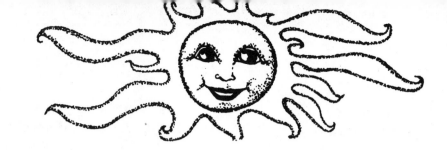

CELERY STUFFED WITH AVOCADO

1 avocado
1/2 C onions, minced
1-2 T lemon juice

4-6 stalks celery

1 t tamari
1 t kelp
1 t basil

Peel and mash the avocado. Mix in the remaining ingredients. Stuff the celery stalks with the mixture. Delicious!

RELISHES

RAW PEPPER RELISH

1 sweet red bell pepper
1 green bell pepper
1/2 C celery
1/2 C cauliflowerettes
1 medium carrot

1/2 medium onion
1/2 C shredded cabbage
4 T soaked and chopped wakame
1 T tamari
1 t each: thyme, basil, kelp

Mince or grate all vegetables. Place in a metal bowl or pail, and pound them with a potato masher, baseball bat, etc. Mash for about 5 minutes, until the juice is set free from some of the vegetables. Tamp the vegetable mixture into glass jars, and cover tightly. Allow the relish to stand, refrigerated, at least 24 hours before using. Keep refrigerated constantly until used. Makes about 3 cups of relish.

Read about Sauerkraut, page 8, for more ideas on how to make relishes, and fermented foods. This relish is an unfermented kind of sauerkraut, basically. Try fermenting it, following the procedures outlined on the sauerkraut pages. You can add different amounts of the vegetables, and any type of firm vegetable.

The more you pound the vegetables, the less firm their texture will be. Try different amounts of pounding and different fermenting times -- from 1 to 7 days.

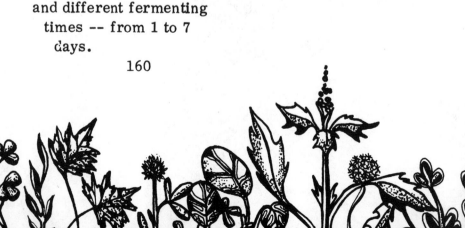

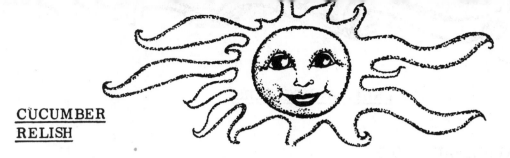

CUCUMBER RELISH

2 large cucumbers
1/3 C chopped parsley, watercress, or mint (or a combination of all three)
1/4 C freshly squeezed lemon juice
2 T water
1 T tamari
1 T honey (optional)

Peel the cucumbers if they are waxed. Dice, or slice very thinly. Mix the chopped greens with the liquids. Pour this mixture over the cucumbers, and allow all to marinate in refrigerator for at least 4 hours before serving. Makes about 3 cups.

ONION RELISH

2 C thinly sliced onions
juice of 1 lemon
1 T honey

Slice the onions very thinly, and place in a jar. Pour the lemon-honey mixture over the onions, and tamp the onions down firmly into the juice, so that they are covered. This will keep, refrigerated, quite a long time (a month or so). It is good to have on hand to add to vegetable salads. The onions lose some of their "bite." For 2 cups.

BEET GARNISH

2 C freshly grated beets   juice of 1 large lemon   1 T honey

Place the beets in a glass jar with a tightly fitting cap. Mix the lemon juice and honey; pour over the beets. Tamp the beets down into the marinade, making sure they are covered. Refrigerate a day before eating. Will keep about a month. For 2 cups.

Try this with other vegetables -- broccoli, cauliflower, potatoes, corn.

161

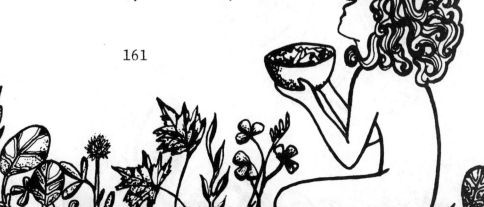

FRUIT APPETIZERS

UNCOOKED APPLESAUCE DIP

3 large organic apples   1/2 C apple juice or rejuvelac   6 pitted dates

Core and dice the apples, leaving the peel on. Pour the rejuvelac into the blender, and drop in the apple pieces and the dates. Pour this into a serving bowl and surround with a platter of fruit pieces speared with toothpicks -- nectarine chunks, pear and apple pieces, pitted cherries, peach slices, blueberries, fresh apricots.

Enjoy this with a summertime fruit salad dinner. Three large apples will make about 2 1/2 cups of sauce.

FILLED APPLE DISCS

3 apples, cored   1/4 C almonds, chopped
3-4 dates, pitted and cut up   1/2 C hazel nuts, chopped
3-4 dried figs, pitted and cut up   1/2 C raisins, soaked

Grind all but apples together in a hand grinder, or chop all ingredients well, and mix together by hand. Form into long rolls and allow them to sit in the refrigerator or freezer for a few hours to set. Core apples. Cut into saucer-like slices, and place on a tray. Cut the dried fruit roll into similar round slices about 1/3"-1/2" thick. Set the dried fruit disc onto the apple slice and press down slightly, and shape at the same time to form a round circle in the center. Save a few almond pieces to top the discs. Makes about 2 dozen.

FRUIT PLATTER

3 cups any fruit soup or the Uncooked Applesauce Dip
1 1/2 quarts fruit pieces

Surround the dip with the fruit pieces; serve with toothpicks.

NUT BUTTERS

ANY NUT BUTTER

1 1/2 C nuts (ground to a meal, or chopped)
2-4 T coconut oil
1 t tamari (optional)

Put the oil in the blender. Add in nuts slowly, and process until you achieve the consistency you desire -- smooth, or crunch. Use a rubber spatula to keep the nuts flowing into the blades. This makes about 1 cup.

Try different nut combinations -- sunflower/cashew, almond/sesame -- the possibilities are endless! The amount of oil you will need will depend upon the oil content of the nut you use. Black walnuts, pecans, filberts, brazil nuts, almonds, cashews all have a high oil content and will require less oil.

TAHINI

1 1/2 C sesame seed, or sesame seed meal
2-4 T   coconut oil
1 t tamari

Put oil and tamari in blender, and slowly add in seeds. Add in oil as needed for a thick, heavy consistency.   For 1 cup.

ALMOND/CASHEW BUTTER

1 C almond meal
1 C cashew meal
4-5 T coconut oil
1 t tamari

Put 3 T of oil in the blender,
and while motor is running,
pour in the nut meal. Add
oil and meal bit by bit,
keeping a smooth tex-
ture. 1 1/2 cups.

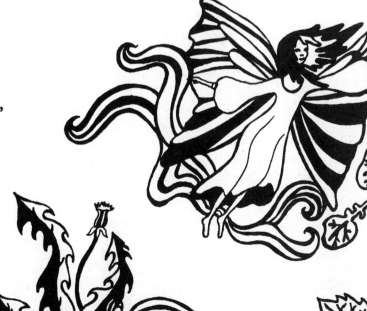

163

APPENDIX I
GLOSSARY

BLACKSTRAP MOLASSES   A natural sweetner made from raw sugar cane

BLENDING   Using a blender to reduce food from solid to liquid state. Best
  method: Put liquid in blender <u>first</u>, then add in fruit or vegetable
  pieces while motor is running. Process as little as possible, on
  lowest possible speed to retain maximum nutritive value.

BRONNER'S SEASONING   A commercial organic vegetable seasoning.

BUCKWHEAT LETTUCE   A 7-day-old indoor green grown from unhulled buckwheat
  seed, and rich in lecithin and vitamins. Excellent as a salad base.

CAROB   Chocolately tasting powder made out of ground pods from the evergreen
  leguminous tree <u>Ceratonia carrubia</u>. High in the minerals calcium,
  potassium and phosphorus. 3 T carob powder and 2 T water = 1 square
  chocolate.

CHAPATIS   Living bread made from homogenized, soaked wheatberries.

COCONUT OIL   Oil extracted from fresh coconut and recommended for use whenever
  oil is indicated. (See page 21)

DULSE   A red seaweed, <u>Rhodymedia palmata</u>, which contains many trace minerals.
  Used as a seasoning.

ENZYME   A substance found in all living things which helps bring about chemical
  changes. Fermented foods are full of enzymes.

ESSENE BREAD   Bread wafer made through "baking" ground wheatberries in the
  sun or on top of a radiator.

FERMENTATION   The breakdown of complex molecules in living foods caused by
  the action of a ferment such as bacteria or yeast.

FERMENTED NUT/SEED or PROTEIN SAUCE   Another name for seed sauce.

GRAIN CRISP.   A crisp bread "dried" in a dehydrator.

GREEN DRINK   Chlorophyll drink made from greens.

GREEN ONIONS   Another name for scallions.

GRIND   For seeds or nuts, to reduce to a fine powder or meal. Use a hand
  grain mill, blender, electric nut/seed grinder, or run through Champion
  juicer with homogenizing plate in.

HIZIKI See Sea Vegetable.

HOMOGENIZE To reduce to the same fine consistency. When referring to vegetables means to blend well, or run through meat grinder, food grinder or Champion juicer with homogenizing plate in.

INDOOR GREENS Buckwheat lettuce and sunflower greens. See pages 16 - 18.

JUICING To extract the liquid from fruits or vegetables, leaving the pulp.

JUNIPER BERRIES The bitter blue-black or purple berries of the coniferous ever-green shrub or tree, Juniperus communis. Used as a sauerkraut seasoning.

KELP Seaweeds high in iodine and other minerals. A good salt substitute, generally powdered. See Sea Vegetables.

LACTOBACILLUS ACIDOPHILUS Bacteria found in fermented foods which promotes good digestion and growth of intestinal flora.

LIVE FOODS Unprocessed, uncooked natural foods still containing the "breath of life."

LIVING BREAD Chapatis or Essene bread.

PIGNOLIAS Pine nuts.

PROTEIN LOAF Another name for seed loaf.

REJUVELAC Fermented beverage made from soaking soft white pastry wheat. The water of Hippocrates Health Institute. See page 6.

SAUERKRAUT One of the three main fermented foods served at Hippocrates. High in digestion-aiding enzymes, lactic acid, and vitamins C and K. See page 8.

SEA VEGETABLES Sea weeds or vegetables: arame, wakame, nori, dulse, kombu, To use: soak at leat 10-20 minutes, then cut with scissors. Also can be crumbled and used dry as a salad garnish. High in trace minerals and iodine.

SEED MILK   1 part seed : 3 parts liquid.
    SAUCE   1 part seed : 2 parts rejuvelac. Ferment 4-8 hours.
    CHEESE 1 part seed : 1 part rejuvelac. Ferment 8-12 hours.
    LOAF   6 parts seed : 1 part rejuvelac. Ferment 24-48 hours.

SEED MEAL Ground seed.

SEED YOGHURT Seed cheese.

SOAK WATER Residual water from soaking dried fruits, sprouts or nuts; used as a base for dressings and sauces.

SPROUTS New growth of any seed. Those most frequently used at Hippocrates are: alfalfa, chick pea, fenugreek, lentil, mung, radish and sunflower.

SUNFLOWER GREENS One of the two 7-day indoor greens. Grown from unhulled sunflower seeds. An excellent salad base.

TAHINI Sesame seeds ground into a thick, buttery paste. Sesame seed butter.

TAMARI Seasoning sauce made from fermented soybeans. High salt content.

TRITICALE A 50/50 mixture of 1 1/2 - 2 day-old sprouted wheat and rye.

VEGETABLE SAUCE Any vegetable combination blended to sauce consistency. See pages

VEGETABLE SEASONING A ground natural food seasoning. Commercial varieties include Dr. Brunner's, or try Joseph's Seasoning, page 37.

VITAMIN Any of the accessory food-factors found in many foodstuffs that perform specific tasks essential for normal growth.

WHEAT, HARD RED WINTER Used for wheatgrass and sprouting.

WHEAT, SOFT WHITE PASTRY Used for making rejuvelac.

WHEATBERRIES Wheat kernels.

WHEATGRASS JUICE A chlorophyll drink extracted from wheatgrass. Rich in vitamins and minerals.

WHEATGRASS JUICER Hand juicer that extracts juice from greens without oxidation.

APPENDIX II

SALAD INGREDIENTS

LEAFY VEGETABLES
(GREENS)

argula
asparagus
beet greens
bok choy
brussel sprouts
buckwheat lettuce
burdock leaves
cabbage
    chinese or celery
    green
    red
    savoy
    white
cardoon
celery
    green
    white
chayote leaves
chicory leaves
chickweed
clover leaves
collards
comfrey leaves
curly dock
dandelion greens
endive
    curly endive or chicory endive
    escarole or broad leaf endive
    french or belgian endive
fennel (anise)
fiddleheads (young fern shoots)
garden cress
kale
kohlrabi leaves (turnip cabbage)
lambsquarters
lettuce
    bibb
    boston or butterhead

lettuce
    bibb
    boston or butterhead
    iceberg or cabbage
    leaf
    oakleaf
    red leaf
    romaine or cos
mustard greens
mustard-spinach
nasturtium leaves
parsley
plantain
pokeweed
purslane
radish greens
rhubarb
sorrel
spinach
sunflower greens
swiss chard
turnip greens
watercress
white mustard
wild lettuce
winter cress

FLOWER
VEGETABLES

artichokes, globe
broccoli
cauliflower

SALAD INGREDIENTS

WILD EDIBLES (GREENS)

burdock leaves
chickweed
chicory
clover
comfrey
curly dock
dandelion leaves
fiddleheads
lambsquarters
nasturtium leaves
plantain
pokeweed
purslane
sorrel
watercress
wild lettuce
winter cress

ROOT VEGETABLES (TUBERS)

artichoke, jerusalem
beets
burdock root
carrot
celeriac (celery root)
horseradish
kohlrabi
parsnips
potatoes
   white
   sweet (yams)
radish
rutabaga
salsify (oyster plant)
turnips

Bulbs

garlic
leeks
onions
  Bermuda
  button
  green (scallions)
  Italian
  Spanish
  white
  yellow
shallots

FRUITS OF THE VINE
SUCCULENT VEGETABLES

beans,
  green
  wax
cucumbers
eggplant
okra
peppers
  red
  green
pumpkin
summer squash
  cocozelle
  cymling
  crooked neck
  straight neck
  chayote
  vegetable marrow
  pattypan
  zucchini
winter squash
  buttercup or turban
  butternut
  acorn
  golden delicious
  hubbard

ADDITIONAL SALAD INGREDIENTS

avocado
chives
fresh corn off the cob
green lima beans
mushrooms
fresh peas
  green
  snow pea pods
sprouts
tomatoes

SEES

SALAD OILS

TO EAT

sesame
sunflower
pumpkin

FOR SEASONING

anise
caraway
celery
coriander
cumin

dill
fennel
flaxseed
mustard
poppy

FOR SPROUTING

(see chart, page 13)

cabbage
fenugreek
garlic
lettuce
mustard
onion
parsley
radish
   red, white
   black
red clover
sesame
sunflower
squash

almond
avocado
brazil nut
cashew
coconut
corn
cottonseed
filbert
oat
olive
peanut
pecan
pistachio
rice bran
rye germ
safflower
sesame
sorghum
soybean
sunflower

NUTS

acorns
almonds
brazil nuts
cashews
chestnuts
coconut
filbert

hickory
macademia
peanut
pecans
pignolias (pine nuts)
pistachios
walnuts

FRUITS

ACID FRUITS

Berries:
   blackberries
   cranberries
   gooseberries
   raspberries
   strawberries
Citrus:
   grapefruit
   lemon
   lime
   orange
   tangerine, tangelo
Currants (fresh)
Kumquat
Pineapple
Plum
Pomegranate
Ugli

SUB-ACID FRUITS

Apple, fresh
Apricot
Blueberry
Cherry
Fig, fresh
Grape
Huckleberry
Kiwi
Mango
Nectarine
Papaya
Peach, fresh
Pear, fresh
Quince

SWEET FRUITS

Banana
Dried fruit (all)
   currants
   dates   apples
   figs   peaches
   prunes   pears
   raisins

MELONS

casaba   honeydew
cantaloupe   muskmelon
crenshaw   sugar
    watermelon

Avocado combines with acid and sub-acid fruits.

169

INDEX

CORRECT FOOD COMBINING

PROTEINS
<POOR>
STARCHES

PROTEINS
NUTS
*CEREALS (WHOLE GRAINS)
*DRIED BEANS & PEAS
OLIVES
DAIRY FOODS
FLESH FOODS
SEA FOODS

STARCHES
POTATOES
*CEREALS (WHOLE GRAINS)
* DRIED BEANS & PEAS
JERUSALEM ARTICHOKES
HUBBARD SQUASH
PUMPKIN
CHESTNUTS

<GOOD>

GREEN VEGETABLES

<GOOD>

EXCEPT NUTS WITH ACID FRUITS POOR

POOR

POOR

POOR

FRUITS

FRUITS

ACID <FAIR> SUB-ACID <FAIR> SWEET

ACID
CITRUS FRUITS
PINEAPPLES
PLUMS (SOUR)
POMEGRANATES
STRAWBERRIES
SOUR FRUITS
ETC.

SUB-ACID
APPLES
APRICOTS
CHERRIES
GRAPES
MANGOES
PAPAYAS
PEARS, ETC.

SWEET
BANANAS
DATES
FIGS
PRUNES
RAISINS
PERSIMMONS
ETC.

◄—— POOR ——►

AVOCADO – BEST WITH ACID OR SUB-ACID FRUIT OR GREEN VEGETABLES

TOMATOES – MAY BE TAKEN WITH NON-STARCHY VEGETABLES AND PROTEIN

MELONS — EAT THEM ALONE OR LEAVE THEM ALONE

*THESE FOODS ARE SOURCES OF BOTH PROTEINS AND STARCHES.

GENERAL FOOD COMBINING

The most basic and fundamental idea about food combining is: let your body be your guide. The chart opposite presents optimum, and general food combinations, but each person is in a different stage of balance. Each person has a different, unique constitution: each has had a different history, a different series of foods to take in and absorb; a different set of circumstances in which all these factors played; no two people are at exactly the same place, but every person can take these ideas, and apply them usefully.

So, become aware of these ideas, apply them, and see what effects you can sense.

For the most optimum digestion, eat every food alone, separately and independently. Each food has its own rate of digestion and absorbtion, and your body is set up to handle one food at a time. For variety though, we mix our foods, and, due to this physiological set-up, it's very important to see what similar foods mix well together, and why dissimilar foods don't.

From the chart below, you can see, basically, what foods break down where. Try to combine foods that break down in the same area of the body. If you mix, for example, a dense, highly concentrated sunflower seed (which is broken down in the stomach), with a lighter food, such as an orange, the orange will get held up in the stomach with the seeds: it will start to ferment, cause gas. It is actually rotting in your system before your system is able to absorb it (in the small intestines). Try to think of putting together foods that can pass along together harmoniously. The combinations outlined on the following page do just that.

PROTEINS	stomach	polypeptides	duodenum	amino acids
STARCHES	mouth	polysaccarides	duodenum	simple sugars
FATS	duodenum	fatty acids		

When you enjoy a food, try and see if you can eat the whole, complete food: the beet greens along with the beet roots, the celery leaves as well as the stalk, and the peel as well as the more tender inner portions. Nature provides complete foods that your body can break down, even though they contain a variety of compounds: proteins as well as starches, and sometimes fats.

Some basic guidelines are: eat fruits independently from vegetables. Fruits and vegetables do not combine. When eating fruits, enjoy melons separately. Melons are broken down very rapidly, so enjoy them as a separate group. Leafy greens combine well with just about every other vegetable, and are an aid to digestion.

The best teacher of all, as always, is your own body. Your body can handle more extreme combinations, perhaps, than can another's. When on a cleansing diet, follow these guidelines for improved health; follow them daily for continued good health and ease in digestion.